Jin Shin Healing

"This book is very practical and easy to use! All the healing flows are well illustrated and quick to apply. I also appreciate the positive and encouraging way in which the author deals with the topics of life. Just reading this book makes me feel good. I often use the finger holds of Jin Shin Jyutsu to fall asleep, which is an enormous help to me. As a natural therapist I also recommend this book to my clients."

— BETTINA VON NOTTBECK, natural therapist and trauma therapist

"I've been using Jin Shin healing touch for just over one year. I find the main central flow exercise most helpful for balancing and awakening my energies in the morning. It's a great way to begin the day! I also benefit from using holds and touches for specific issues on an 'as needed' basis. I found the book to be a clear, concise, and easy reference. In my view, Jin Shin and similar meridian treatments may be our best friend in times of emergency."

— MARCUS LINDNER, mindfulness practitioner, Findhorn Community

Jin Shin Healing Touch
Quick Help for Common Ailments

Tina Stümpfig

Translated by Karen Lüdtke

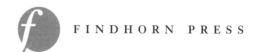

FINDHORN PRESS

Findhorn Press
One Park Street
Rochester, Vermont 05767
www.findhornpress.com

Findhorn Press is a division of Inner Traditions International

Disclaimer
The information in this book is given in good faith and is neither intended to diagnose
any physical or mental condition nor to serve as a substitute for informed medical
advice or care. Please contact your health professional for medical advice and treatment.
Neither author nor publisher can be held liable by any person for any loss or damage
whatsoever which may arise from the use of this book or any of the information therein.

Cataloging-in-Publication Data for this title is available from the Library of Congress

ISBN 978-1-64411-076-8 (print)
ISBN 978-1-64411-077-5 (ebook)

Printed and bound in the United States by Versa Press, Inc.

10 9 8 7 6 5 4 3 2 1

Edited by Jacqui Lewis
Cover images: www.dreamstime.com
Text design and layout by Damian Keenan
This book was typeset in Adobe Garamond Pro, Calluna Sans,
with Editor Condensed and Alana Plus used as a display typefaces

To send correspondence to the author of this book, mail a first-class letter to the
author c/o Inner Traditions • Bear & Company, One Park Street, Rochester,
VT05767, USA, and we will forward the communication, or contact the author directly
at **www.harmonie-der-mitte.de**

Contents

Preface

This book provides you with a special kind of medicine cabinet for which you need neither specific remedies nor any kind of essence, but solely and exclusively your hands.

The method of Jin Shin Jyutsu described here is ancient but nonetheless highly current. It is the art of bringing life energy into harmony, increasing our vitality and joy in life and strengthening our self-healing capacities.

And it is yet more: it is a form of intuitive knowledge that we all carry within us from birth and unconsciously use time and again. When you rest your head in your hands, you are harmonizing points on your head that help you to remember things. When you cross your arms, you are activating certain points in the crook of the elbows that help you stand in your power and authority. Maybe as a kid at school you always sat on your hands? This strengthened your concentration and memory. Babies who suck their thumbs are harmonizing their digestive systems. They are also calming and comforting themselves when feeling insecure in a still new and often frightening world. When you put your hand on your shoulder, tension and stress are released. You also free yourself from the burdens that you have accumulated over the course of your life and carried around as a matter of course.

As such, we automatically use the art of Jin Shin Jyutsu consistently without being aware of it. How wonderful it is to make conscious use of this ancient knowledge to strengthen and harmonize ourselves, simply by placing our hands on certain points on our body—thereby allowing many physical, psychological and spiritual issues to simply dissolve!

This book invites you to use this simple and effortless art and to experience its gentle healing power first-hand.

1

The Healing Art of Jin Shin Jyutsu

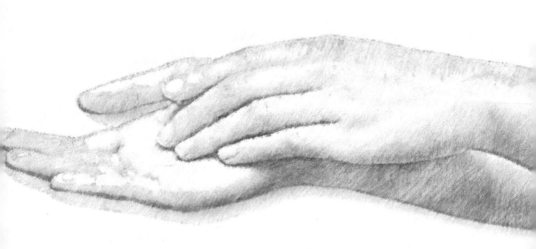

Introduction

What Is Jin Shin Jyutsu?

Jin Shin Jyutsu—colloquially also simply referred to as "Jin Shin"—is an ancient source of knowledge about the harmonization of life energy. It is said to have been spread all over the world hundreds of years ago and to have been transmitted orally from generation to generation until eventually it was forgotten and used only intuitively, if at all.

Jiro Murai from Japan rediscovered and researched this gentle art of self-healing at the beginning of the twentieth century, following his own recovery from a very serious illness. He transcribed his knowledge and passed it on to his students Kato Sensei and Mary Burmeister. As a result, this art was given a Japanese name: Jin Shin Jyutsu, which translates as the "Creator's art through the compassionate person".

Jin: knowing, compassionate person
Shin: creator
Jyutsu: art

Mary Burmeister introduced the art of Jin Shin Jyutsu to the Western world and hence made it accessible to us once again.

Jin Shin Jyutsu is a gentle healing art that you can use on yourself and of course also on other people, as well as animals. By placing your hands on certain points on the body, life energy is harmonized and restored to a vibrant flow. As self-healing capacities are mobilized, body, mind and soul become geared towards healing and complaints and symptoms are alleviated or completely eliminated.

You can use Jin Shin Jyutsu in parallel to any other therapies, even if you are receiving medical treatment. Jin Shin Jyutsu treatments can, for example, reduce the side effects of medication and reinforce and speed up recovery following surgery. Jin Shin Jyutsu is not a miracle cure, but an art for harmonizing life energy in the body. Yet, miracles can happen, especially if you deeply engage and trust yourself.

Health, vitality and well-being depend on the free and even distribution of life energy in the body. When life energy flows harmoniously, human beings are healthy. When there are blockages in the energy pathways that bring life into the body, these become manifest relatively quickly through disharmony, discomfort and the first symptoms of disease. If energy remains imbalanced, these symptoms become consolidated, more severe or chronic, and may even lead to new symptoms.

Jin Shin Jyutsu works with 26 so-called safety energy locks, which lie on each side of the body and are arranged symmetrically to the spine. These are points on the body where energy is available in a highly concentrated form and where, simply by holding these points, blockages can easily be released. By placing your hands on particular safety energy locks—depending on the subject or symptom—you bring yourself back into harmony spiritually, mentally and physically, blockages are released, symptoms dissolve, and gradually—or sometimes even quite suddenly—you are filled with new life force, vitality, joy, serenity and trust.

The Application of Jin Shin Jyutsu

Place your fingertips, fingers or palms on the points indicated until life energy begins to flow freely again. With a little practice, you will be able to feel this. It is noticeable as a slight tingling, pulsating or flowing—hence the term "flow". However, different people may experience this in a slightly different way.

You need to do nothing other than hold these points. You do not remove anything and you do not add anything. Your hands simply serve, so to speak, as jumper cables, so that life energy can flow strongly and consistently again, while empty energy batteries can recharge themselves. You will probably not sense this flow or pulsation at first; in our everyday life we are not used to paying attention to such subtle energies, so it may take a while for you to attune to these.

Until then, simply keep to the following basic rules:

- Maintain each hold for 3–5 minutes, then move on to the next one.
- If you only do one hold, feel free to maintain it for 15–20 minutes.
- For a longer flow, such as the main central flow with its seven steps, take about 30 minutes for the entire sequence, which comes to about 4minutes for each hold.
- Only harmonize energy points for as long as it feels enjoyable and comfortable.
- When it gets tiring, switch to another hold or take a break.
- If some points are difficult to reach, just hold other points; there are always different options.
- And if you have problems reaching the energy locks on your feet, the substitute for all energy locks on the feet is safety energy lock SEL 15 (p. 32) in the groin area!

You can treat yourself as often and for as long as feels good.

When you treat others, roughly keep to the following times:

- Adults: not more than one hour at a time
- Children: infants no more than 20 minutes, older children no more than 40 minutes at a time
- Babies: just a few minutes
- Elderly or very sick people: not more than half an hour at a time
- Animals: 10–30 minutes (animals usually show you when they have had enough by turning away or simply walking off)

What matters is that all this is effortless and—even if it sounds a bit strange —that you do not hold any intention in mind. Needless to say, when you are sick, you obviously want to change this, but change can most easily come if, as mentioned before, your hands simply act as jumper cables without your thoughts and expectations getting in the way of the energy flow.

Brief instructions for harmonizing energy points:

- First and foremost: it needs to be relaxed and effortless!
- You do not do anything: you simply hold the various points and thereby automatically jump-start life energy, in order for it to flow freely and strongly again.

- First apply the holds as described. If you find something too tiring, hold another point or vary the holds by not crossing your arms or by swapping your hands. The indicated holds are possibilities. You decide what points you hold and what is best for you.
- You can do the holds first on one side and then on the other side of the body. You can also just treat one side, depending on what you like and what feels best.
- Maintain each hold until you feel energy flowing strongly again—if you do not notice this shift, do not worry as it does not affect the treatment or its effect. Just follow the time indications on p. 15.
- Assume an attitude of receiving. You do not have to do anything—other than to simply be. Let your hands rest on the indicated energy locks and allow yourself to receive the ever-increasing flow of energy with your entire being.

Helpful Hints

Relax!

Jin Shin Jyutsu is effortless—release all strains and struggles. Pay attention to what is good for you. Do not focus your attention on the issues or symptoms that you have, nor on getting rid of them. Instead notice the inner harmony, the life energy, the pulse of life, that is ALWAYS there no matter how great the imbalance may be—we would not be alive if this pulse did not exist. By way of holding different points you strengthen this pulse. What we pay attention to is strengthened. That is why we talk about projects rather than problems when harmonizing energy points.

You can do something with a project, something can come of it, change is possible, whereas with problems we easily get stuck and then see only the problem. If, while giving a treatment, you find yourself reflecting—being without thoughts would of course be great, but let's face it: who can do that for any length of time?!—then think in possibilities and solutions rather than problems.

And stick with the inner question: How can this get even better?

You cannot go wrong! Let your intuition guide you and find your own personal path. Simply lay your hands on the energy locks you have selected and just let things happen. Life energy finds its way—trust it. Once again, as it is so important: you cannot go wrong. There are no wrong points or holds. Harmonizing energy points is always linked to the intelligence of the body, and even if you apply a "wrong" hold, nothing bad happens. The body turns things around the way it needs them to be, and it simply takes a little longer for the desired effect to kick in.

Keep Going!

In the case of severe imbalances, with serious or chronic illnesses, it is especially important to harmonize energy points regularly. This is because blockages or unhealthy patterns will have developed over years or even decades. Regular treatment can reinforce the once-healthy pathways to such an extent that all blockages can be released and harmonious patterns can reassert themselves—permanently.

Jin Shin Jyutsu is not about "removing" symptoms—even though certain holds are assigned to certain symptoms—but rather about restoring perfect balance. Rather than fighting against bothersome ailments, the entire body system is gradually harmonized again. Rather than repairing the body, we bring it back into alignment.

Regular treatments allow you to drop into a deep state of physical, mental and spiritual relaxation, thanks to which comprehensive regeneration and healing can take place.

Be Patient!

Do not let yourself be intimidated if at first you notice no change with respect to a particular issue that you are treating. Harmonizing energy points always works—but sometimes the initial impact is not what you would expect or wish for. Our bodies always begin by regulating what is most urgently needed, whatever is most indispensable in a given moment.

However, this does not mean that harmonizing energy points can replace a doctor. Go for a check-up if you feel unwell. You can always treat yourself in addition to any medical care. Holding points strengthens the immune system, supports the healing of wounds and regeneration, e.g., after surgery, and also harmonizes any side effects, if you need to take medication.

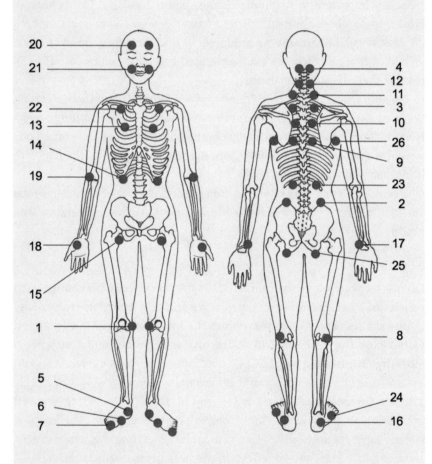

The 26 Energy Locks

The 26 Energy Locks –
Gateways to Heaven

The safety energy locks or SELs, also simply known as "energy locks", are, as mentioned, specific points on the body where energy is highly concentrated. When touched, these points pass on the stimulus they receive, setting in motion a great deal, as they lie on the energy pathways that bring life into the body. Blockages that develop on these pathways interrupt energy flows and ultimately upset the entire energy flow pattern in a given area.

These give rise to disharmony and disease. The safety energy locks—hence the name—also act as an early warning system for the body. When certain areas are overloaded, they serve as circuit breakers—they shut down to stop imbalances affecting the entire body. As such, they also point to the origin of an imbalance and by holding the respective energy locks this imbalance or blockage can be released again. This is why the energy locks are also known as Gateways to the Kingdom of Heaven.

Each energy lock has a specific meaning and is related to body, mind and soul. When you place your hands on the respective energy lock, blockages are released, energy regains momentum and spiritual, psychological and physical impairments can be dissolved again.

The 26 energy locks are symmetrically located along the spine on each side of the body.

Each lock is approximately palm-sized (or, in animals, the size of one of their paws or hoofs), i.e., if you know a lock's approximate location, you cannot miss it.

For some energy locks we also use a high or low point. This is located about a hand's breadth above or below the respective energy lock.

You will find the location and use of each of the 26 energy locks in detail on the following pages.

SEL 1 promotes deep and easy exhalation; helps with breathing and letting go; supports renewal and change; ensures inner stability; releases stress; clears the head; promotes self-esteem and self-confidence; helps us to step into action/motion, to express our abilities, to be authentic and to recognize solutions and possibilities; harmonizes the skin; helps digestion.

SEL 1 is located on the insides of the knees.

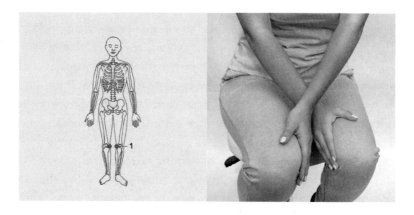

High SEL 1 is located about a hand's breadth above SEL 1, on the insides of the thighs.

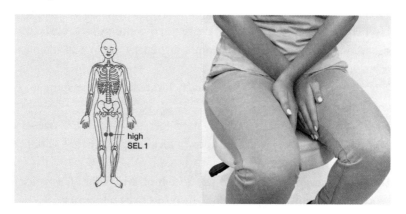

SEL 2 promotes inhalation and readiness to receive; strengthens our life force; helps us walk tall through life; acts as a personal chiropractor; gives structure to life; evokes confidence; helps with despair, competitiveness, fear of not being good enough, sadness, melancholy, tension, stress, exhaustion, fatigue, dizziness and high blood pressure.

SEL 2 is located on the back at the upper edge of the pelvic rim.

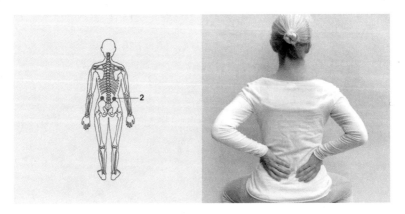

SEL 3 promotes understanding; is the door that swings open so that tensions can be discharged and purified energy and new vitality can be received; facilitates stepping into action; helps us to see things from different perspectives and to be able to meet life challenges with ease; releases stress; helps to let go of doubt and expectations; harmonizes the immune system; aids with colds, flu and allergies.

SEL 3 is located on the back between the upper corner of the shoulder blade and the spine.

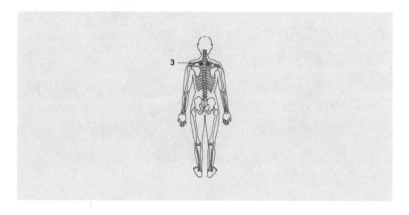

Since you cannot hold both SELs 3 in a relaxed way, it is recommended instead to hold SEL 3 with SEL 15.

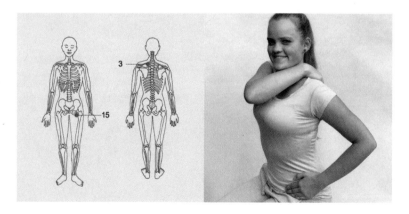

SEL 4 is a window allowing in the breath of life; helps to manifest visions; releases fears and doubts; evokes deep trust; an important energy lock for anxiety and depression; calming; helps us to switch off; promotes new perspectives; helps with insomnia, eye and ear issues; first aid point for unconsciousness, shock etc.

SEL 4 is located on the neck at the base of the skull.

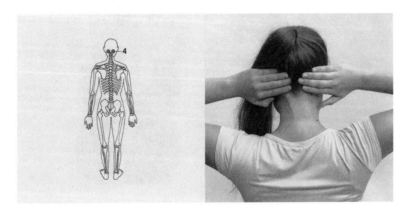

SEL 5 personal psychologist; promotes renewal; helps with letting go; releases fears, uncertainty and doubts; strengthens our intuition, will to live and vitality; promotes impartiality; helps to discard old thoughts and habits; frees us from self-imposed limitations; harmonizes ears.

SEL 5 is located on the inside of the ankle between the ankle bone and heel.

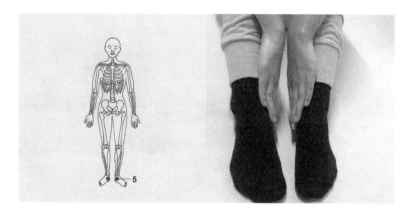

SEL 16 supports SEL 5, so you can also hold the two energy locks together.

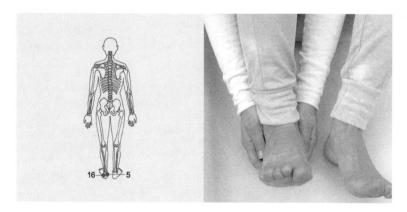

SEL 6 promotes emotional and physical balance; helps us to be sincere and authentic; releases tensions in the back, shoulders, pelvis and hips; personal chiropractor.

SEL 6 is located on the arch of the foot.

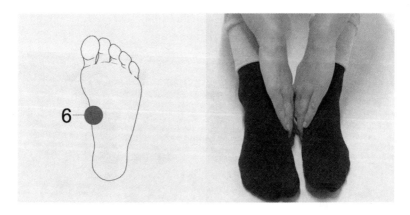

SEL 15 supports SEL 6, so you can also hold the two energy locks together.

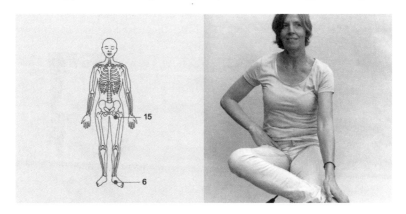

SEL 7 strengthens vitality; helps us let go of anything that obstructs us and makes success difficult; promotes clarity; connects thinking and feeling; supports us to release debilitating habits; strengthens patience with ourselves, joy and ease; relieves stress and tension in the head, back and hips; first aid point for unconsciousness, shock etc.

SEL 7 is underneath the big toe.

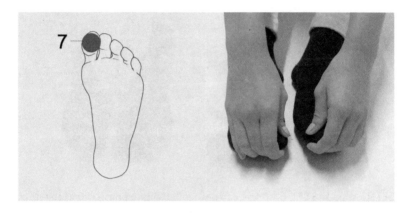

To open SEL 7, you can also hold SEL 2 together with SEL 15.

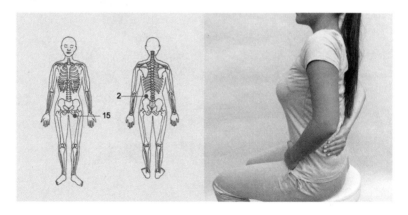

SEL 8 supports the interconnection of opposites; connects us with the rhythm, strength and peace of the universe; helps us accept ourselves; strengthens trust; encourages constructive rage and anger management; promotes inner serenity and peace; helps us discover life's infinite possibilities; harmonizes muscles and skin; regulates body temperature; helps with tooth and jaw issues; harmonizes all assimilatory and excretory functions of the body.

SEL 8 is located on the outside of the back of the knee.

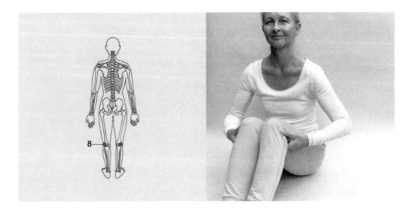

The **low SEL 8** is located on the outside of the calf about a hand's breadth below SEL 8.

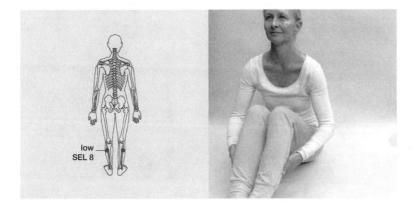

SEL 9 helps with completion of the old and with new beginnings; ensures clarity; supports the release of worries, tension and stress; stops thoughts going round in circles; harmonizes rage, anger, irritability and frustration; lets us move forward with joy and ease; harmonizes liver and gall bladder; helps with all feet-related issues.

SEL 9 is located on the back between the lower corner of the shoulder blade and the spine.

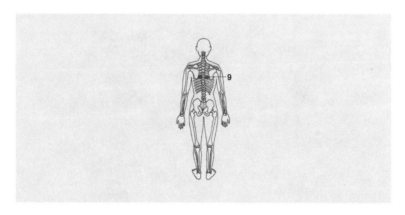

Since it is difficult to hold this energy lock on yourself with ease, the substitute point for this lock is **SEL 19** in the crook of the elbow.

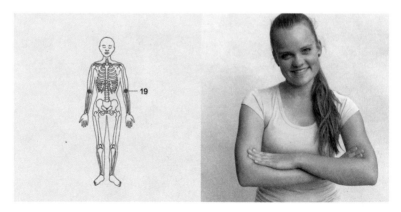

SEL 10 helps us see abundance rather than lack; supports mental clarity; calms emotions; brings about vitality, self-awareness, peace of mind and serenity; enables us to recognize interrelationships; helps to allow feelings; dissolves effort; harmonizes circulation and blood pressure; strengthens the immune system.

SEL 10 is located on the back above SEL 9 between the middle of the shoulder blade and the spine.

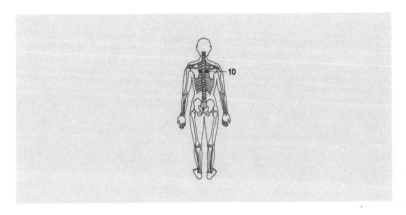

Here again there is a substitute point for self-help, namely the high SEL 19, which is located on the inside of the upper arm about a hand's breadth above SEL 19.

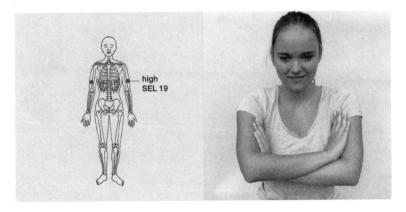

SEL 11 supports letting go of excess baggage (like taking a heavy backpack off the shoulders); promotes balance and harmony; resolves fears, sadness and negative thinking; enhances ease; helps with decision-making and letting go of guilt; harmonizes shoulders, neck, head, hips and legs; helps with preventing stroke and high blood pressure.

SEL 11 is located at the top of the shoulder.

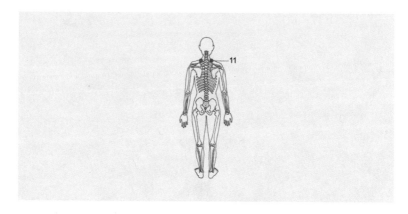

Holding both SELs 11 together is rather uncomfortable, so it is best to hold SEL 11 together with SEL 15.

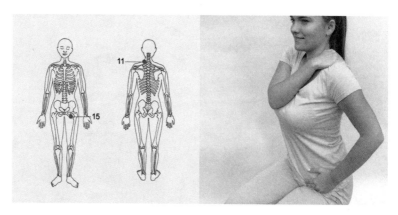

SEL 12 connects us with the one universal source; strengthens primal trust; resolves fears and depression; restores emotional balance; facilitates our experience of belonging to the whole again; releases tensions in the arms, neck and shoulders.

SEL 12 is located in the middle of the neck next to the cervical spine.

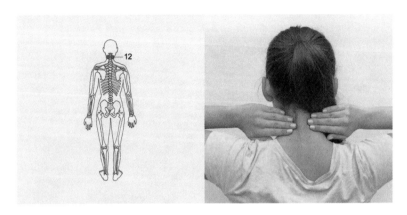

SEL 13 helps with transitions; promotes inner and outer growth, creativity, renewal, self-acceptance and self-love; facilitates creativity; supports the transformation of consciousness; helps us to love even our "enemies" or people who seem hostile (also what seems hostile within ourselves); assists with taking on responsibility; helps with disappointment and frustration; harmonizes mood swings; stabilizes the endocrine and immune systems; helps with addictions; beneficial for all serious illnesses.

SEL 13 lies on the chest just below the third rib.

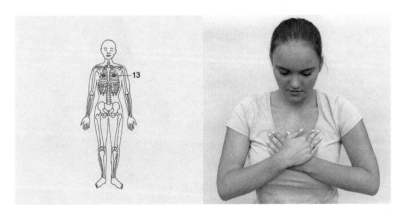

SEL 14 strengthens our awareness of being connected to heaven and earth; indicates what needs to be well nourished on all levels; promotes (primal) trust; helps to digest everything (physically and emotionally); resolves envy, jealousy, competitiveness, deprivation, rage, anger and worry; harmonizes sleep; ensures inner stability; helps with heartburn, bloating and stomach ache.

SEL 14 is located on the abdomen below the last rib arch.

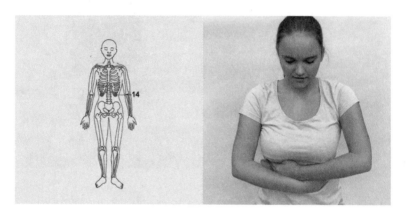

SEL 15 brings joy, laughter, happiness and lightness to life; supports the healing of all wounds and injuries (visible and invisible); promotes clear thinking, peace of mind and vitality; evokes courage, strength and a deep sense of safety; helps with stress and exhaustion; lets us live from the heart; an important SEL for the time before and after surgeries.

SEL 15 is located in the groin area.

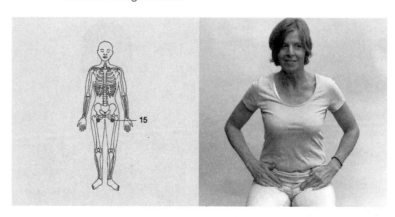

SEL 16 helps to release rigid patterns and habits; heals old scars; harmonizes fears and insecurities; allows us to move forward to break new ground with joy and enthusiasm; resolves paralysis and rigidity; sets us in motion; strengthens connective tissue; harmonizes teeth, gums, jaws and bones.

SEL 16 is located on the outside of the ankle between the ankle bone and heel.

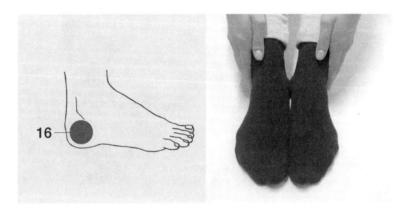

SEL 8 supports SEL 16, so you can hold the two energy locks together.

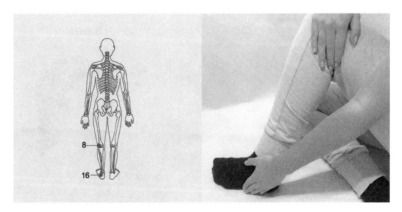

SEL 17 brings the mind to rest; stops thoughts from going round in circles; releases tension and stress; provides access to our intuition and creative power; is supportive in cases of straining and effort; helps with exhaustion; harmonizes the nervous system; helps with shakiness and fainting.

SEL 17 is located on the outside of the wrist on the little-finger side.

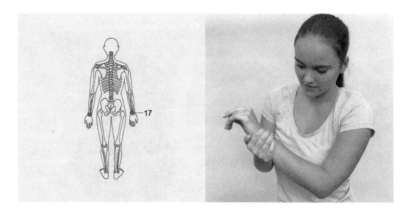

SEL 18 helps us let go; strengthens trust; harmonizes thinking/the mind; promotes sound sleep; good for all sleep issues.

SEL 18 is located on the inside of the hand on the ball of the thumb.

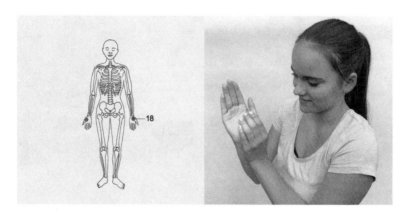

SEL 19 strengthens our inner authority and awareness; gives us strength to persevere; helps to maintain balance even in crisis situations; connects us with the source of all life; strengthens self-love and self-esteem; harmonizes tinnitus, ringing in the ears and allergies.

SEL 19 is located in the crook of the arm on the side of the thumb.

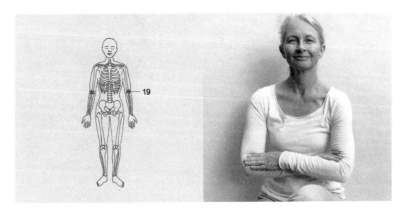

The high SEL 19 is located on the inside of the upper arm about a hand's breadth above SEL 19.

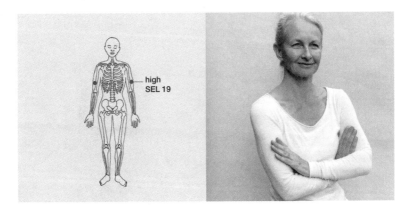

SEL 20 connects us to the flow of life; strengthens inner knowledge, mental clarity and intuition; gives new strength; harmonizes headaches, migraines and blood pressure.

SEL 20 lies on the forehead above the eyebrow.

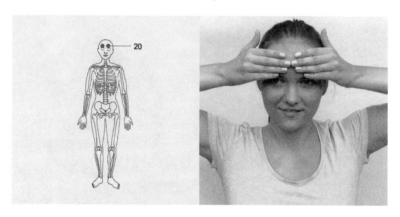

SEL 21 conveys a deep sense of safety and confidence in life; lets us look beyond our own limitations; gives energy and wakes us up; helps us take on responsibility; supports us to let go of the "burdens of the world"; harmonizes colds, sinusitis, toothache and neuralgic pain.

SEL 21 lies below the cheekbone.

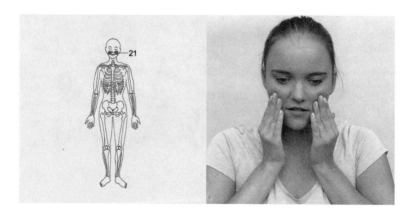

You can also hold SEL 21 together with SEL 22, as these energy locks support each other.

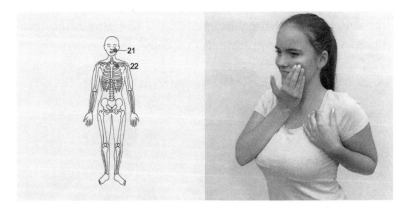

SEL 22 supports loving acceptance; helps us adapt in a positive way (to situations, circumstances and environmental stimuli/poisons that we cannot currently change); strengthens our openness to new things; allows us to see new paths and possibilities, and to rediscover our zest for life; helps with anxiety and panic attacks; brings about a deep understanding of the world and ourselves; harmonizes thyroid gland, parathyroid gland and lymphatic flow.

SEL 22 lies under the collarbone.

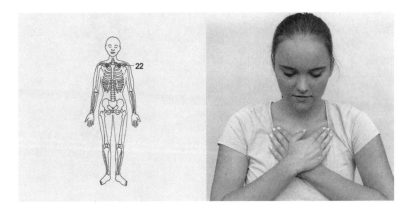

SEL 23 important energy lock to transform fear; enables us to change our lifestyles, so we can live our potential; promotes clear thinking, awareness of interconnections and stress reduction; strengthens trust (in ourselves), courage and patience; harmonizes addictions; strengthens the immune system; cleans, detoxifies and deacidifies the body.

SEL 23 is located on the back below the last rib arch.

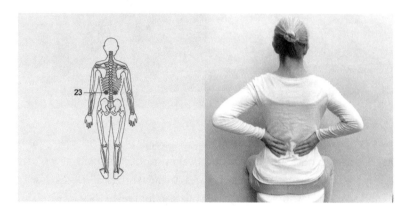

You can also hold **SEL 23** together with **SEL 21** as both energy locks support each other.

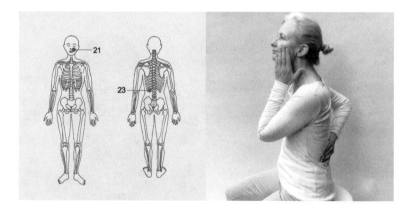

SEL 24 solves chaos and confusion; brings peace to mind and body; provides a deep understanding of ourselves and others; helps with exhaustion and shakiness.

SEL 24 is located on the outside of the foot about halfway between the little toe and heel.

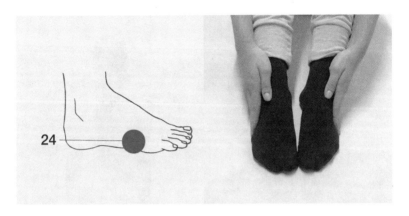

You can also hold **SEL 24** together with **SEL 26** as both energy locks support each other.

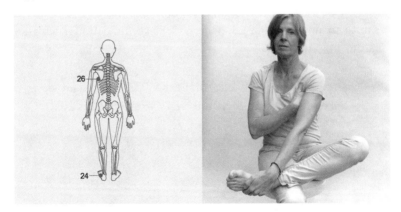

SEL 25 promotes recovery, regeneration and renewal; gives new strength; relaxes; promotes clear thinking, alertness and concentration; provides body, mind and soul with new energy; harmonizes metabolism; has a detoxifying and diuretic effect.

SEL 25 is located at the lower end of the sitting bone. You can hold both SELs 25 by simply sitting on your hands.

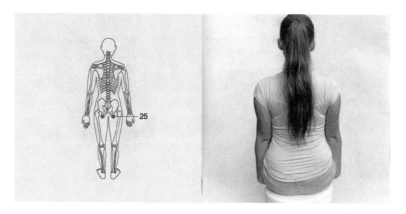

SEL 26 helps us to be present in the moment; brings about inner peace, awareness, a deep sense of being cared for and safe, vitality and equilibrium; allows us to see new possibilities; helps with all accumulations such as cysts, tumors and growths.

SEL 26 is located on the outer edge of the shoulder blade. When you practise the big hug (p. 41), you automatically hold both SELs 26.

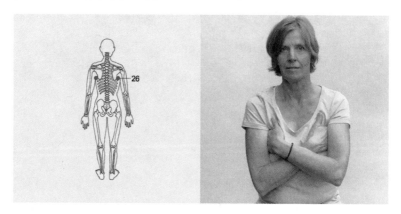

General Harmonizers

General harmonizers are holds or flows that you can use at any time, as they have a very comprehensive effect. Hence, they are described in detail right at the beginning of this book and then repeatedly referred to with respect to different themes and symptoms.

The Big Hug – Connecting to the Great Breath of Life

The "36 conscious breaths", as Mary Burmeister called them, make up a very simple and powerful flow. It is also called the "big hug", as you literally embrace yourself.

This exercise takes only about 5 minutes, depending on how fast you breathe. Use it to calm down, when you feel stressed, to regain strength, when the monotony of daily life has you too firmly in its grip or when you are insecure or anxious.

- Sit comfortably, cross your arms and put your hands under your armpits with your thumbs pointing upwards—give yourself a hug.
- Loosen your shoulders while your head is relaxed and slightly tilted forward.
- Take a deep breath in and out again.

Mary Burmeister always said the following to introduce this exercise:

- "Be the dropping of your shoulders and exhale all dust, dirt and greasy grime."
- Then start counting your breaths: Inhale—exhale (1)—inhale—exhale (2). Count to 36.
- You do not need to focus on breathing in any particularly deep or drawn-out way; just breathe as usual—or better still, let yourself be breathed by life—in and out—in and out ...
- As you count your breaths, you are helping yourself stay present. You are treating yourself, so to speak, with a pause for reflection. Healing only takes place in the here and now.

- Just be the dropping of your shoulders and let yourself be breathed by life—in and out, in and out—while your whole body relaxes by itself.
- When disturbing thoughts arise, do not pay any attention to them—keep your focus on your breath and let your attitude be one of gratitude.

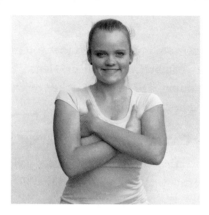

Why is it precisely 36 breaths? Numbers play an important role in Jin Shin Jyutsu: each number has a specific meaning and a specific vibration and is linked to certain themes. Number 36 stands for wholeness, for the ocean sky within which everything is contained, from which we came and to which we will return. We are always connected to it. We receive power and energy from it. It is what nourishes, carries and heals us. Mary Burmeister said that everything was contained in the 36 conscious breaths and they were enough to off-load whatever we burdened ourselves with each day.

The Fingers – Quick Support

Holding your fingers is the easiest way to use Jin Shin Jyutsu. Several energy pathways, which are connected to the entire body, begin and end in each finger. By holding the fingers you harmonize your thinking and feeling, mental and physical fatigue disappears and blockages dissolve, all of which contribute to healing.

Hold each finger for at least 3 minutes. Each finger is associated with a particular emotion—or, as Mary Burmeister put it, attitude:

- **The thumb** harmonizes the attitude of "worry". Holding your thumb releases concerns and brings serenity, trust and inner certainty.

- **The index finger** harmonizes the attitude of "fear". Fear turns into deep trust, love and safety.

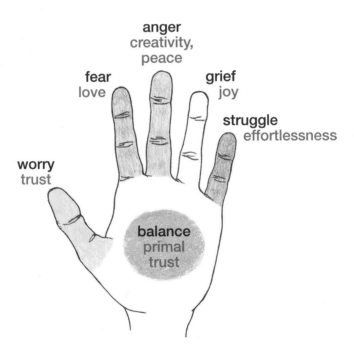

- **The middle finger** harmonizes the attitude of "anger". Anger becomes understanding, inner peace and generosity. You regain access to the full potential of your creativity.

- **The ring finger** harmonizes the attitude of "grief, sadness". It brings about acceptance and strengthens our sense of inner joy.

- **The little finger** harmonizes the attitude of "effort, struggle" and "pretence". Patience and effortlessness emerge out of effort and struggle, while pretence turns into self-love, appreciation and zest for life.

The palm harmonizes the attitude of "despair". It gives you the primal trust you have longed for and brings about relaxation, balance and vitality.

- Loosely hold the individual fingers of your left hand or the left palm with your right hand and then use your left hand to hold the individual fingers of your right hand or right palm. Or just hold the finger that you particularly need.

- **You can hold your fingers whenever you have your hands free:** waiting to pay at the checkout (to stave off frustration about the long queue), talking to friends or waiting at the traffic lights.

- **Even if you have only one hand free, you can hold your fingers:** form a ring with your thumb and the finger you want to hold by placing the tip of the thumb on the nail of the other finger.

- **Further connections between the fingers and related physical and emotional issues and organ function energies:** The organ-function energies are the energies that form, feed and maintain the function of the individual organs. However, in their effect they reach far beyond the respective organs.

44

The Thumb

Attitude: worry; organ function energy: stomach and spleen energy

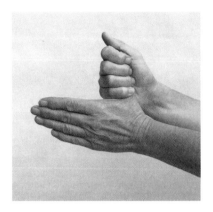

- clarifies and harmonizes from head to toe;
- "windscreen wiper for the mind": harmonizes thinking; stops thoughts going round in circles; helps us get out of negative thought-loops;
- helps us to keep calm in any situation;
- resolves worries and brooding thoughts;
- helps us to love ourselves and others and to feel loved;
- releases feelings of inferiority, fears of missing out, envy and greed; is beneficial if struggling with holding boundaries/taking care of yourself;
- supports us to let go of feelings of lack and to see abundance in life;
- gives mental and emotional clarity;
- helps with nightmares and sleep issues;
- relaxes and releases stress;
- serves people who are consistently late or always in a rush;
- supports us to move calmly and confidently through crises;
- provides a "thicker skin" and strengthens the nerves;
- helps with all addictions and eating disorders;
- strengthens the ability to make decisions;
- helps with everything that has to do with the skin's surface; smooths the skin and gives it a healthy glow;
- helps with everything related to teeth, gums, jaws, nose, mouth and ears;
- harmonizes the digestive organs;
- strengthens and harmonizes stomach and spleen;
- helps with hair loss and strengthens hair growth;
- and supports hormonal balance.

The Index Finger

Attitude: fear; organ function energy: kidney and bladder energy

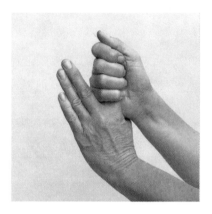

- helps to regain balance;
- helps to reduce fears and insecurities;
- strengthens self-esteem;
- gives confidence and a sense of safety;
- helps to be in the here and now (even with those who live too much in the past or future, or want nothing to do with the past);
- harmonizes melancholy and depression and strengthens the will to live;
- is beneficial for addictions;
- brings about deep regeneration and transformation;
- helps with all pain; removes pain from the body;
- clears the head;
- harmonizes the breath;
- relieves physical tension (neck, back, hip, thigh, knee, calf);
- helps the muscles;
- supports arteries and veins;
- and strengthens and harmonizes the bladder and kidneys.

The Middle Finger

Attitude: rage, anger; organ function energy: liver and gallbladder energy

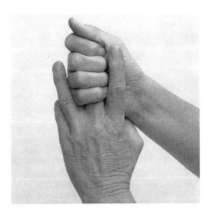

- harmonizes rage, anger and irritability;
- helps us to see clearly;
- harmonizes thinking;
- brings renewal on all levels;
- strengthens creativity;
- assists us to realize ideas and projects;
- helps to consciously shape our life;
- supports us to step into action;
- facilitates new beginnings;
- provides courage and strength to continue in times of crisis;
- is THE finger for all workaholics;
- supports back, hips and pelvis;
- loosens muscles and tendons and supports joints;
- helps with shoulder and neck tension and migraine;
- helps with everything that has to do with the eyes;
- and strengthens and harmonizes liver and gall bladder.

The Ring Finger

Attitude: grief, sadness; organ function energy: lung and large intestine energy

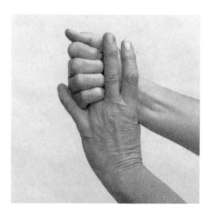

- harmonizes grief and sadness;
- helps to process grief;
- strengthens clear thinking;
- promotes vitality and wisdom;
- relaxes mind and nerves;
- harmonizes feelings of guilt;
- helps with self-pity and hypersensitivity;
- gives us courage to let go of the old and to start something new;
- releases thought and behavioural patterns that are old and outdated;
- transforms problems into projects (revealing new possibilities);
- helps with anything to do with the arms;
- strengthens the voice;
- helps with coughing, hoarseness, bronchitis and sore throat;
- and harmonizes lung and large intestine.

The Little Finger

Attitude: effort, pretence; organ function energy: heart and small-intestine energy

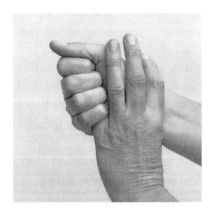

- helps with letting go;
- strengthens willpower;
- supports when nothing inspires you;
- brings deep and true joy and enthusiasm;
- strengthens our zest for life; vitality and love;
- helps us live from the heart and listen to our inner voice;
- assists us in understanding interdependent relationships and to act accordingly;
- brings about effortlessness; peace of mind and serenity;
- strengthens the ability to concentrate and think clearly;
- helps with forgetfulness;
- supports with stress management;
- helps with tendencies to excessive perfectionism and over-analysis;
- is helpful if you always do things you do not want to do;
- has a calming effect on those suffering from sleep disorders;
- supports anything to do with the ears and hearing;
- relieves neck complaints;
- and helps with shoulder, upper arm and elbow conditions.

The Finger–Toe Flow – A Helper in Time of Need

The finger–toe flow is less suited to self-care, as it is very uncomfortable to use on yourself. However, the potency of this flow means that it definitely belongs in the Jin Shin Jyutsu medicine cabinet. If necessary, ask someone else to treat you.

This flow purifies and renews the whole body and helps it heal. Hence, it is often called the "hospital flow". It also flows through all the vertebrae and spinal discs and can offer effective pain relief in cases of slipped discs. It supports all joints and promotes the healing of broken bones and all other injuries. What is more, it is an important flow for strokes and can also facilitate stroke prevention.

The energy between fingers and toes moves from the thumb on one side of the body to the little toe on the other side, from the index finger on one side of the body to the second smallest toe on the other side of the body, and so on.

Hold the following in turn (or let someone hold this sequence on you):

- left thumb and right little toe,
- left index finger and right second-smallest toe (ring toe),
- left middle finger and right middle toe,
- left ring finger and right second toe,
- and finally left little finger and right big toe.

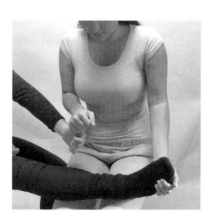

And for the other side of the body hold the following in turn (or let someone hold this sequence on you):

- right thumb and left little toe,
- right index finger and left second-smallest toe (ring toe)
- right middle finger and left middle toe,
- right ring finger and left second toe,
- and finally right little finger and left big toe.

Take 3–5 minutes for each step and hold each until you feel a steady, calm pulsation, or just as long as feels good.

The Main Central Flow –
The Source of Life

The main central flow, also called "main central vertical flow", is the flow that directly connects us with the source of life, our direct line upwards, so to speak. It is the first flow that forms in people and the energy pathway that makes life possible in the first instance. It is the breath of life, or, as Jiro Murai called it, the "great breath of life". The main central flow is our great source of energy, our supply source. It provides us with energy for all body processes and fuels all other flows. It harmonizes the immune system, hormonal system, nervous system, metabolism, cardiovascular system and blood pressure and supports breathing. The main central flow brings new strength and energy to body, mind and soul, and releases fears, stress and depression.

The main central flow consists of seven steps. However, do not let yourself be deterred by the length of the flow. If you use it regularly, you will soon realize how powerful and stabilizing it is. It is most relaxing to lie on your back while using the main central flow, but of course you can also use it while sitting. What matters is that it is comfortable and effortless.

Hold each position for 2–5 minutes.

> **STEP 1:** Place your right hand on the top center of the head, where it will stay until the second last step, and place your left hand on the middle of the forehead between the eyebrows.

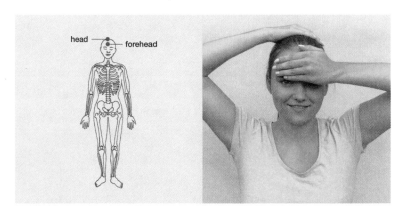

This hold harmonizes thoughts, releases fears and strengthens intuition. It stimulates memory and brain functions and facilitates the prevention of senility and Alzheimer's. It harmonizes the pineal and pituitary glands and stabilizes blood pressure.

52

STEP 2: Place your left hand on the tip of your nose.

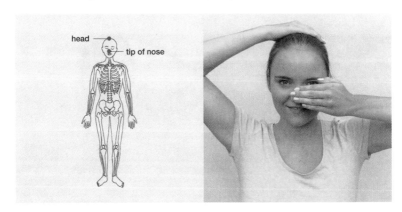

This hold cleanses the sinus cavities, frontal sinuses and maxillary sinuses. It harmonizes the upper half of the body, relieves tension in the pelvic girdle and harmonizes the reproductive organs. It aids the muscular system, supports with all hormonal fluctuations (e.g., puberty, menopause) and helps to see more clearly and to gain new perspectives.

STEP 3: Place your left hand on the pit of the throat, i.e., on the upper end of the sternum.

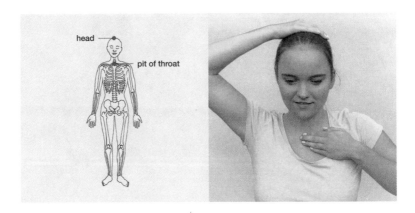

This hold harmonizes the thyroid and parathyroid glands, stimulates metabolism and regulates calcium and magnesium levels. It also stabilizes blood pressure and is important for bone structures. It calms the mind and harmonizes feelings. It also helps us adapt to environmental situations, radiation, air pollution and other stressors (including emotional ones).

STEP 4: Place your left hand on the center of your sternum.

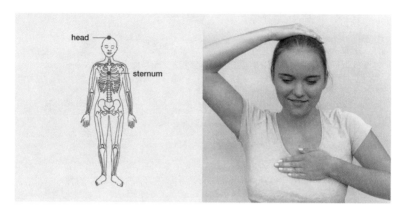

This hold strengthens the thymus, invigorates the immune system and strengthens the heart, circulation and breathing. It opens the heart; it helps us to live from the heart, to release feelings of guilt and of not being good enough, and to love ourselves and others.

STEP 5: Place your left hand on your stomach about three fingers above the belly button.

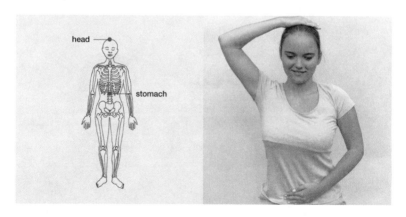

This hold strengthens the stomach, spleen, kidneys and pancreas. It stimulates digestion and supports the immune system. It also harmonizes cell structures and reduces the risk of cancer. It strengthens the cardiovascular system and harmonizes the nervous system. It helps us to relax and release stress, to deal more easily with aggression and to develop deeper trust in life.

STEP 6: Place your left hand on the pubic bone.

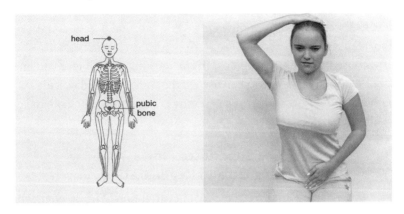

This hold releases tensions in the lower abdomen and legs, harmonizes the reproductive organs, strengthens the spine and spinal discs and regulates digestion and the fluid balance in the body. It calms the mind, gives a deep sense of security and inner safety and stimulates creativity.

STEP 7: Place your right hand on the coccyx, while the left hand remains on the pubic bone.

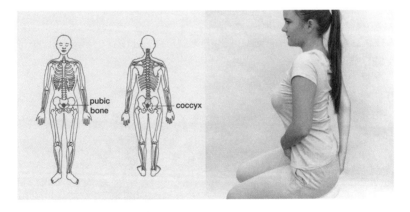

This hold supports blood circulation in the legs and feet. It harmonizes from head to toe, clears thoughts, helps us to think in terms of solutions and possibilities and gives new energy when you feel tired, exhausted and listless.

Each of these steps has its own specific effects, and you can of course use the steps that particularly appeal to you, or touch on certain topics, one at a time. Nevertheless, it is good to use the entire flow, as it addresses everything in one go.

If you use the main central flow in the morning, it will give you energy and momentum for the day. When used in the course of the day, it assists you to both relax and refuel, and in the evening it helps you switch off and get a good night's rest.

The Supervisor Flows –
Letting Go and Regenerating

The supervisor flows arise from the main central flow. The 26 energy locks are located on these flows and, as their name suggests, they supervise the two sides of the body.

These flows help to relieve stress, to release any baggage we carry, to relax, to regenerate and recharge, to be honest and sincere and to be true to ourselves. They enhance our capacity to deal with crises and loss, to better cope with bad memories and to start each day with joy and strength.

The supervisor flows can be used at all times, no matter the symptoms we are dealing with. They always help and harmonize.

For the left supervisor flow:

STEP 1: Place the right hand on the left SEL 11 and the left hand on the left SEL 25.

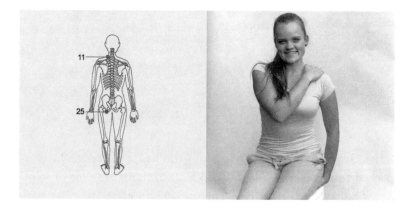

STEP 2: Leave your right hand on the left SEL 11 and place your left hand on the left SEL 15.

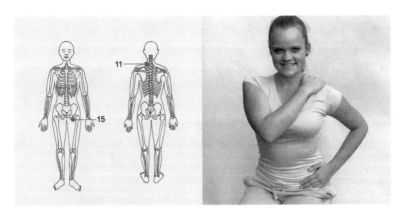

For the right supervisor flow, reverse the holds:

STEP 1: Place the left hand on the right SEL 11 and the right hand on the right SEL 25.

STEP 2: Leave your left hand on the right SEL 11 and place your right hand on the right SEL 15.

The Mediator Flows –
Life Is Movement and Change

The mediator flows harmonize our energy levels and balance out tensions and stress. They mediate between the two supervisor flows when energy is unevenly distributed, interweave the two sides of the body and adjust imbalances, if there is too much or too little energy on one side of the body. The mediator flows are always useful when something has stiffened—physically, mentally or spiritually. These flows dissolve rigidity, help us deal with transitions and change, support us in processing bad experiences or traumas so as not to be crushed by them, move us into action and strengthen our ability to act. They let us breathe freely again and can also help to resolve deep sadness and depression.

The mediator flows can be harmonized with a simple hold.

For the left mediator flow:
Place the right hand on the left SEL 3, behind the left shoulder, so that your fingertips lie between the top of the shoulder blade and the spine. With the left hand form a ring with thumb and ring finger by placing the tip of the thumb on the ring-finger nail. Then bring your knees together as well.

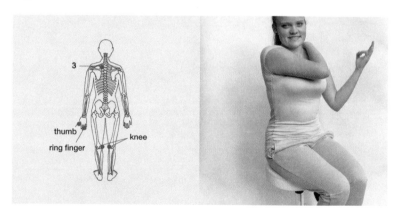

For the right mediator flow:
Place the left hand on the right SEL 3 and use the right hand to form a ring with thumb and ring finger by placing the tip of the thumb on the ring-finger nail. Bring your knees together.

If you find this flow too strenuous to use while sitting down—it is often difficult to keep your knees together with ease—you can use it lying down instead: when you lie on your side and pull up your knees they will connect automatically.

The Spleen Flow – Personal Sunbed

The spleen flow is also called "personal sunbed" or "mini-break". It moves the corners of the mouth upwards, balances feelings and brings joy and lightness.

It flows up the front of the body from the toes, providing life-giving energy to our whole being. It helps recharge used-up energy batteries, opens the solar plexus and nourishes all other flows.

The spleen flow

- provides calm, balance, vitality and new momentum;
- evokes deep trust in life;
- brings about joy and enthusiasm;
- helps with fatigue and lack of energy;
- releases fears;
- evokes a sense of primal trust;
- helps to let go of what is old and useless—including old patterns—so something new can arise;
- releases thoughts of lack; helps us see abundance;
- resolves worries and brooding thoughts;
- helps with all forms of hypersensitivity and low tolerance for frustration;
- brings rhythm to life;
- relieves stress and tension and has a harmonizing effect on all stress disorders;
- supports healthy; restful sleep and also helps with nightmares;
- assists with hypersensitivity, e.g., with regard to noise, bright lights or certain foods;
- harmonizes the nervous system, hormonal system, immune system, cardiovascular system and metabolism;
- helps with allergies and is the most important flow for hay fever;
- aids with the absorption of minerals;
- helps with everything concerning speech, language, voice and vocal cords (slurred speech; extremely soft voice; stuttering; etc.);
- supports keeping the organs in place (in all cases of prolapse);

- strengthens the reproductive organs and is an important flow for the unfulfilled desire to have children;
- aids with Alzheimer's, dementia and Parkinson's;
- helps guarding against cancer;
- has a strengthening effect during chemotherapy;
- helps the nerves;
- supports the thyroid;
- helps with indigestion; bloating and flatulence;
- regulates weight;
- regulates eating disorders;
- harmonizes menstruation (in cases of too much or too little bleeding, irregular periods, cramps);
- and strengthens the connective tissue.

For the left side of the body use the following holds:

STEP 1: Place the left hand on the left SEL 5 and the right hand on the coccyx.

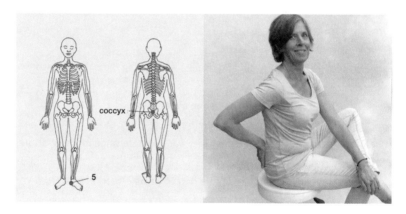

STEP 2: Leave your right hand on the coccyx and place your left hand on the right SEL 14.

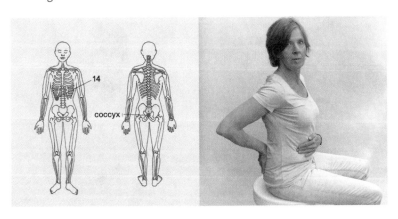

STEP 3: Now leave your left hand on the right SEL 14 and place your right hand on the left SEL 13.

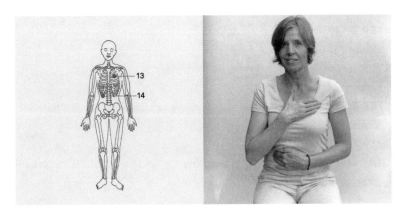

STEP 4: The left hand remains on the right SEL 14 while the right hand moves to the right SEL 22.

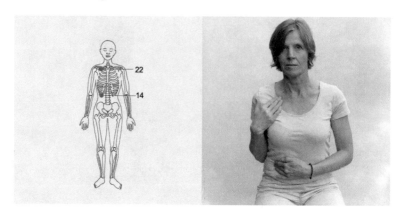

For the right side of the body, reverse the holds:

STEP 1: Place your right hand on the right SEL 5 and your left hand on the coccyx.

STEP 2: Leave your left hand on the coccyx and place your right hand on the left SEL 14.

STEP 3: Now leave your right hand on the left SEL 14 and place your left hand on the right SEL 13.

STEP 4: The right hand remains on the left SEL 14 while the left hand moves to the left SEL 22.

QUICKIE: Use Step 1 of the spleen flow. Or hold both SELs 22 with hands crossed.

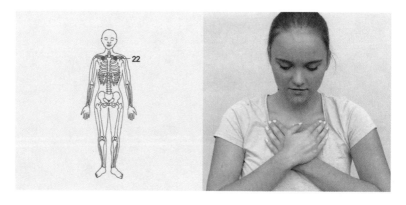

Associated Finger: thumb

The Stomach Flow –
Windscreen Wiper for the Mind

The stomach flow flows from head to toes and, as such, harmonizes from head to feet. It clears the mind and frees up the head. It opens the midriff, so that energy can flow down and back up unhindered again.

The stomach flow

- brings thinking into balance, clears thoughts and stops them from going round in circles;
- frees us from worries and brooding thoughts;
- helps us to love ourselves and to feel loved;
- helps to digest everything—physically, mentally and emotionally;
- resolves feelings of inferiority;
- harmonizes envy, jealousy, greed and the fear of missing out;
- relieves stress and aids those who are always in a rush;
- is good for those who are consistently late;
- harmonizes all kinds of addiction;
- can help control a sweet tooth;
- helps us take on responsibility;
- provides new courage and new perspectives;
- is important for anything to do with the head, i.e., teeth, gums, jaws, sinuses, nose, ears and also headaches;
- harmonizes diarrhea; constipation and flatulence;
- helps with recurring tonsillitis;
- is an important flow for the skin; e.g., acne, skin allergies, excessively dry or greasy skin;
- helps with hair loss and premature grey hair;
- supports the thyroid gland and harmonizes all hormone levels;
- helps with rough, cracked lips;
- harmonizes muscle tone;
- and supports the knees.

For the left side of the body use the following holds:

STEP 1: Place the right hand on the left SEL 21, where it remains for the entire flow, and the left hand on the left SEL 22.

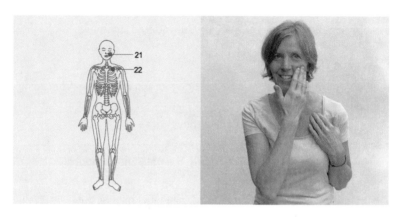

STEP2: Place the left hand on the right SEL 14.

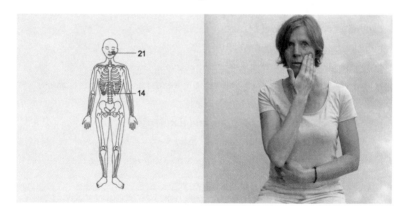

STEP 3: Now place the left hand on the right SEL 23. If it is easier, you can also hold SEL 23 with the back of the hand.

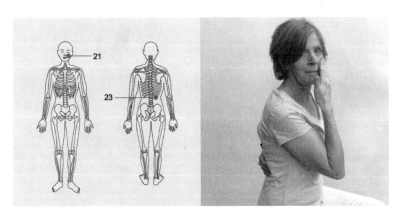

STEP 4: Now the left hand moves to the left SEL 14.

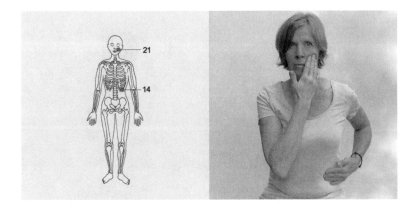

STEP 5: Place the left hand on the right high SEL 1 (on the inner thigh about a hand's breadth above the knee).

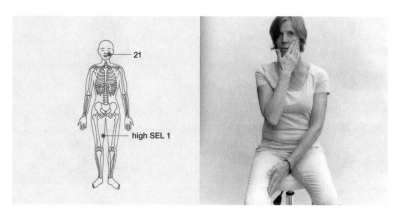

STEP 6: Place the left hand on the right low SEL 8 (on the outside of the calf approximately one hand's breath below the back of the knee).

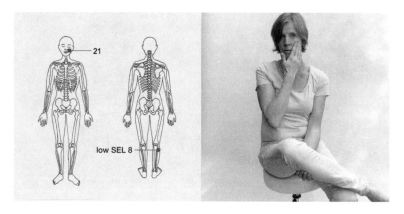

STEP 7: Now hold the right middle toe with the left hand.

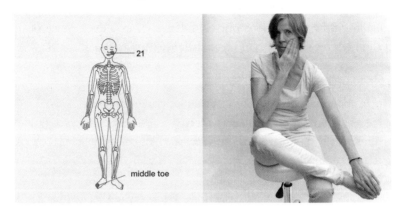

For the right side of the body, reverse the holds:

STEP 1: Place the left hand on the right SEL 21, where it stays, and the right hand on the right SEL 22.

STEP 2: Place the right hand on the left SEL 14.

STEP 3: Place the right hand on the left SEL 23.

STEP 4: Now the right hand moves to the right SEL 14.

STEP 5: Place the right hand on the left high SEL 1 (on the inner thigh about a hand's breadth above the knee).

STEP 6: Place the right hand on the left low SEL 8 (on the outside of the calf approximately one hand's breath below the back of the knee).

STEP 7: Now hold the left middle toe with the right hand.

QUICKIE: Use Step 1 of the stomach flow.
Associated Finger: thumb

The Bladder Flow –
Balancer and Protector

The bladder flow strengthens our confidence, gives a deep sense of inner safety and serenity and helps us regain balance time and again.

The bladder flow

- is an important flow for all fears, panic attacks and phobias;
- has a harmonizing and balancing effect;
- turns problems into opportunities and helps with overwhelming burdens;
- releases arrogance and obstinacy;
- helps us live in the here and now;
- is helpful for bladder infections, bladder weakness and bedwetting;
- helps with runny eyes and blocked tear ducts;
- helps with water retention (edema);
- helps with earache, tinnitus and sudden hearing loss;
- helps with osteoarthritis, arthritis and rheumatic conditions;
- relieves complaints in the areas of the upper head, back of the head, back of the neck and back (and also helps with slipped discs);
- and helps to detox and reduce acidity.

To harmonize the left side of the body, do the following:
STEP 1: Place the right hand on the **left SEL 12**, where it remains throughout the flow, and the left hand on the **coccyx**.

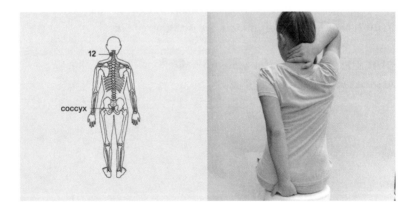

STEP 2: Place the left hand on the hollow of the left knee.

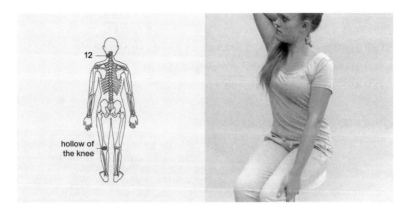

STEP 3: Place the left hand on the left SEL 16.

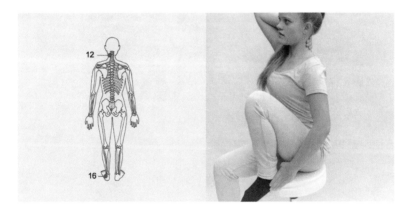

STEP 4: Hold the left little toe with the left hand.

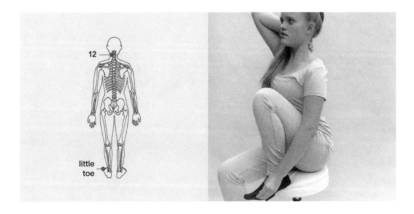

To harmonize the right side of the body, reverse the holds:

STEP 1: Place the left hand on the right SEL 12, where it remains throughout the flow, and the right hand on the coccyx.

STEP 2: Place the right hand on the back of the right knee.

STEP 3: Place the right hand on the right SEL 16.

STEP 4: Hold the right little toe with the right hand.

QUICKIE: Use Step 1 of the bladder flow.

Or just place the hands on the hollows of the knees.

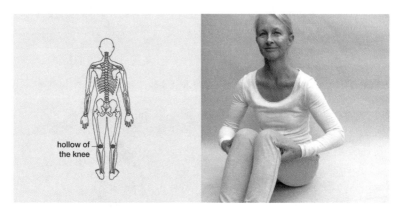

Associated finger: index finger

2

Common Ailments
and Injuries

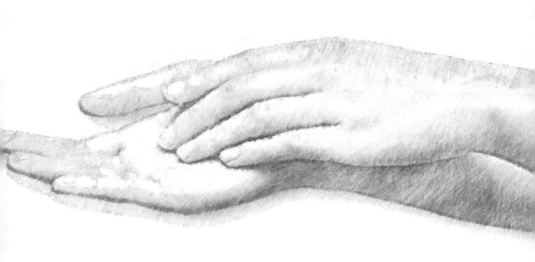

Head

Eyes

For all eye issues (inflammation, defective vision, styes) or for the general strengthening of the eyes:

Place one hand on SEL 20 on the side of the body with the affected eye and the other on SEL 4 on the other side of the body.

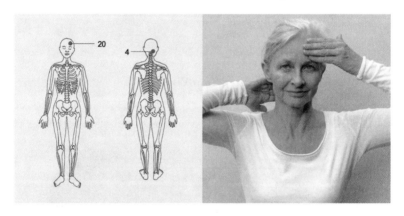

Or place one hand in the armpit on one side of the body and the other hand on the high SEL 19 on the other side of the body.

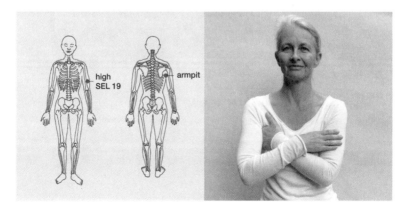

Eye Infection

Use the general hold for the eyes (p. 73).

Or place one hand on SEL 4 on the side of the body with the affected eye and the other on SEL 22 on the other side of the body.

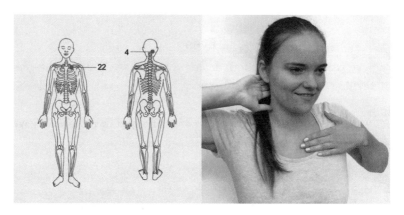

How to Improve and Strengthen Your Vision

Use the general hold for the eyes (p. 73). Or place one hand on the back of the neck on both SELs 4 and the other hand on the chest on both SELs 13.

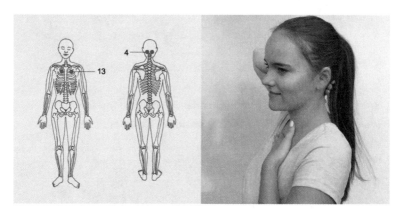

Keep holding your middle finger (p. 47).

Foreign Objects in the Eye

Place your left hand lightly
on the affected eye and
your right hand on top of
the left hand.

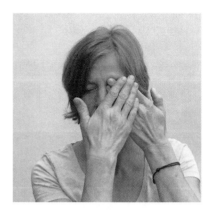

Or hold both SELs 1.

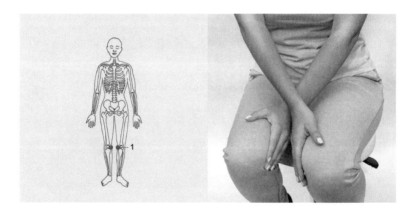

Blocked Tear Ducts

Prolonged tear flow from one or both eyes can be an indication that a tear duct is congested. This is often the case with babies.

To reopen the tear duct, place one hand on the neck between both SELs 12 and the other hand on the coccyx.

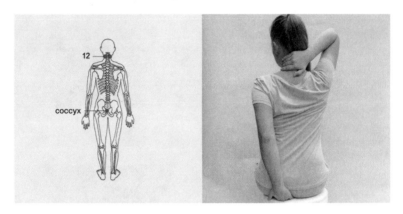

You can also use the bladder flow (p. 68) or step 1 for this.

Ears

The **bladder flow** (p. 68) supports anything to do with the ears and hearing.

As a quickie, you can also place one hand on the back of the neck on both SELs 12 and the other hand on the coccyx.

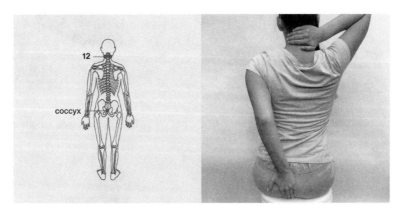

Or hold your index finger (p. 46).

Ear Infection

To relieve pain from ear infections, hold SEL 5 and SEL 16 on the affected side of the body.

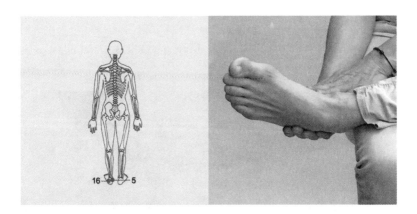

If both ears are affected, you can also treat both sides of the body together by taking one heel in each hand, holding both SELs 5 together with both SELs 16. If this is difficult for you, let someone else treat you.

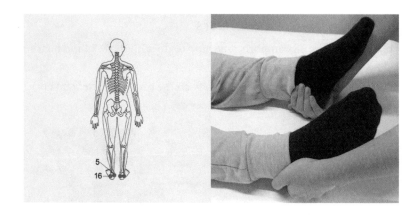

Or place one hand on SEL 13 and the other on SEL 25 on the side of the affected ear.

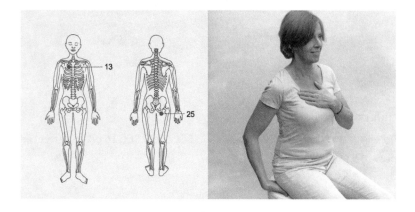

For inflammation of all kinds, you can always hold SEL 3, preferably together with SEL 15.

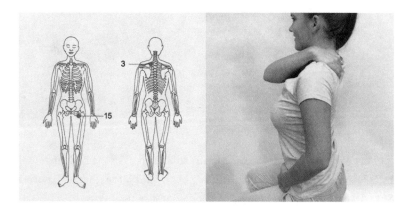

Hearing

If your hearing is impaired, you can use the following holds:

For the right ear:
Place the right hand on the left SEL 11 and the left hand on the right SEL 13.

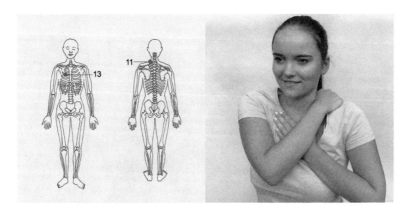

And vice versa for the left ear:
Place the left hand on the right SEL 11 and the right hand on the left SEL 13.

Or place one hand on the pubic bone and with your other hand hold the little toe on the side of the affected ear.

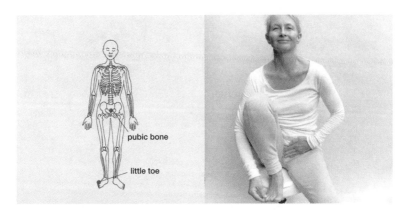

Loss of Hearing

In the case of acute hearing loss, the bladder flow (p. 68) is helpful. Also use the main central flow (p. 52). It helps you to calm down, to return to your true sense of self and to relax. It evokes confidence and serenity.

Or place one hand on the pubic bone and hold both little toes in turn with your other hand.

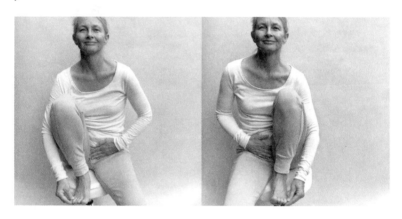

You can also hold both high SELs 1.

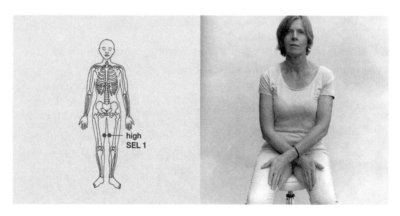

Or place one hand on the forehead on both SELs 20, and the other hand on the back of the neck in the area of both SELs 4 and SELs 12.

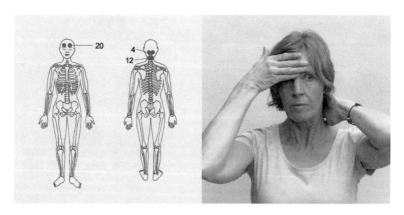

Tinnitus

Tinnitus is a common issue that can be very debilitating. To strengthen yourself overall and to relax, regularly use the main central flow (p. 52).

Also repeatedly hold both high SELs 19.

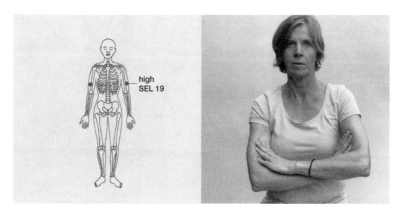

You can also hold SEL 5 together with SEL 15 on the affected side of the body.

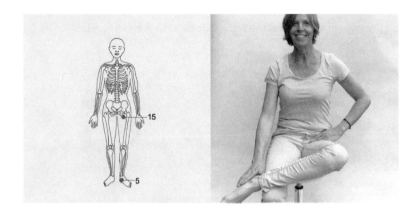

Or place one hand on the pubic bone and hold both little toes in turn with the other hand (p. 80).

To support the right ear:
Place the right hand on the left SEL 11 and the left hand on the right SEL 13.

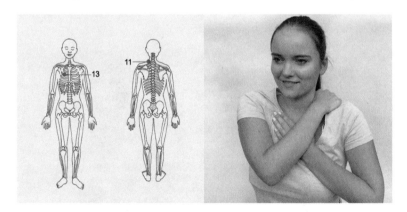

And vice versa for the left ear:
Place the left hand on the right SEL 11 and the right hand on the left SEL 13.

Mouth and Teeth

The stomach flow is suitable for anything to do with the mouth, teeth, gums and jaws (p. 63).

Tooth Decay

To prevent tooth decay, a healthy diet is of course a prerequisite!

You can use the following quickies to strengthen your teeth:
Place one hand on SEL 21 and the other on SEL 22 on the affected side of the body.

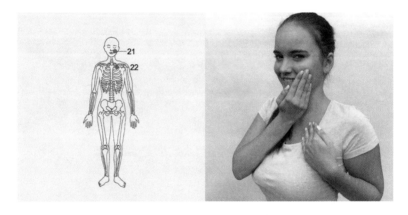

Or hold SEL 16 together with the low SEL 8 on the unaffected side of the body.

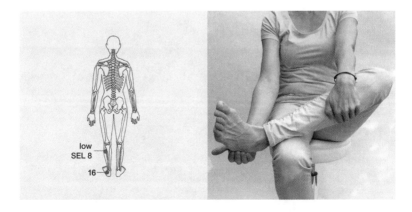

Toothache

To bridge the time until your dentist appointment, you can use the holds for tooth decay (p. 83) and relieve pain by holding SEL 5 and SEL 16 (p. 24).

Gum Issues

Regularly use the stomach flow (p. 63) or just step 1.
Or hold SEL 5 and SEL 16 with one hand and the low SEL 8 with the other hand—both on the unaffected side of the body.

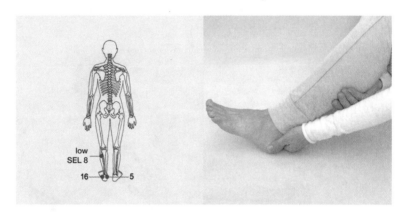

Root Infection

Place one hand over the inflamed area and use your other hand to hold SEL 5 and SEL 16 on the other side of the body.

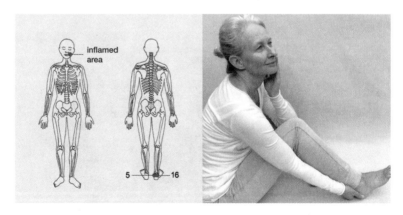

Teeth Grinding

Hold both SELs 14 with your arms crossed.

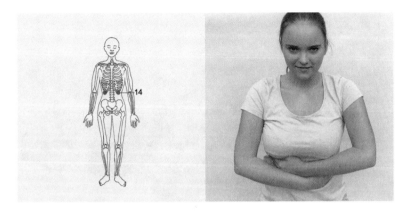

Or hold SEL 14 together with SEL 12.

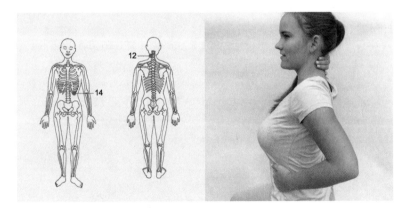

Teething

For the left side of the body:

With just one hand hold the left SEL 5, the left SEL 16 and the left low SEL 8.

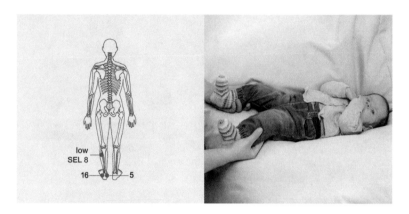

For the right side of the body:

With just one hand hold the right SEL 5, the right SEL 16 and the right low SEL 8.

You can also first, with one hand, hold the heel (SEL 5 and SEL 16) and with the other hand the low SEL 8 on one side of the body. Then reverse the hand holds on the other side of the body.

Brain

Meningitis

Meningitis is a serious illness and always requires prompt medical attention. You can support the healing process with Jin Shin Jyutsu by using the following flow sequences:

STEP 1: Hold SEL 5 and SEL 16 with one hand and SEL 7 on the underside of the big toe with the other hand.

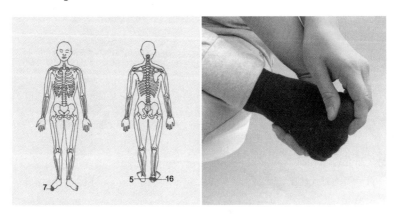

STEP 2: One hand stays on SEL 5 and SEL 16, and with the other hand hold SEL 3.

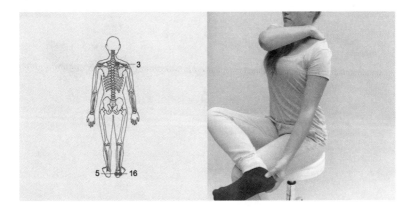

Complete the sequence first on one side of the body and then on the other side.

Stroke

For rehabilitation after a stroke, it is very valuable to use the finger–toe flow (p. 50) on a daily basis. If you yourself are affected, let someone else treat you.

As often as possible, hold SEL 7, either on its own or together with SEL 6.

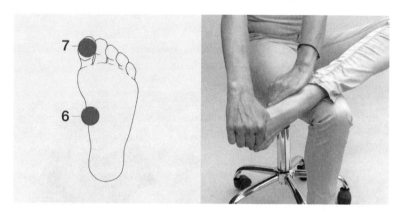

The following flow sequence is also very supportive:
On the unaffected side of the body, hold the following SELs in the order indicated:

STEP 1: SEL 5 and SEL 16.

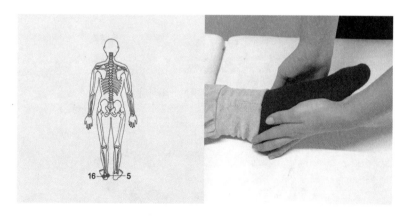

STEP 2: SEL 5 and SEL 15.

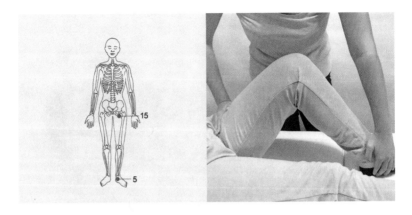

STEP 3: SEL 5 and SEL 23.

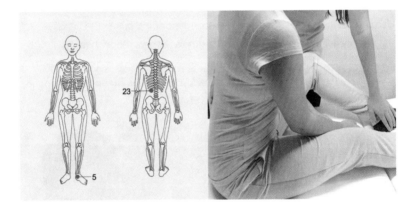

Headaches and Migraine

Headaches and migraines can have different triggers in different people, especially if they occur frequently. Therefore, it is important to look at what the overall, underlying issue might be and to treat it accordingly.

The following are direct treatment aids:

Hold your heels or let them be held: SEL 5 together with SEL 16 is a very helpful hold for all types of pain (p. 157).

Hold both SELs 7 on the underside of the big toes (p. 26).

SEL 1 can also resolve a headache (p. 20).
Hold both SELs 20 (p. 36) or place one hand on the forehead on both SELs 20 and the other hand on the back of the neck on both SELs 4.

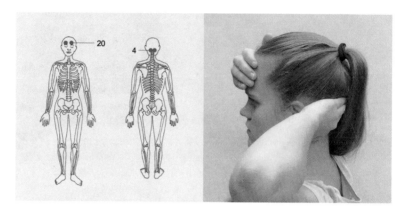

Use the stomach flow (p. 63) or the corresponding quickie—this releases the energy accumulated in the head and discharges it downwards.

If you have pain in the back of your head, practise the bladder flow (p. 68) or the corresponding quickie, or hold SEL 18.

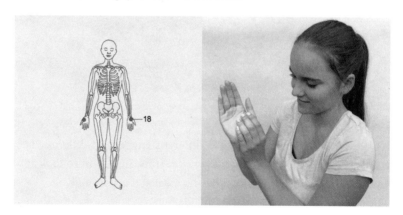

Respiratory Tracts

Upper Respiratory Tract

Cold, Flu, and Fever

An important energy lock for anything to do with viruses or bacteria is SEL3. It is, so to speak, the door that opens to release old, consumed energy and to receive new, purified energy. Viruses and bacteria are always present, but if this door is closed, they cannot leave the body and instead accumulate further.

An important hold for all flu infections is the following:

Place one hand on SEL 3 and the other on SEL 15, first on one side of the body and then on the other side.

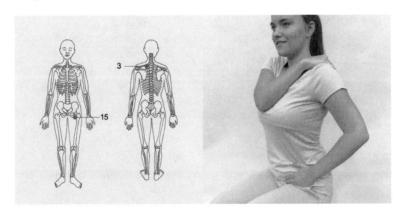

You can also use a flow sequence with several finger holds as depicted on the following page—often it will nip a cold in the bud, so that it does not break out in the first place.

Place one hand on **SEL 3**, and with the other hand, first of all form a ring with **thumb and index finger** by placing the tip of the thumb on the nail of the index finger, then form a ring with **thumb and middle finger**, then with thumb and ring finger and finally with **thumb and little finger**.

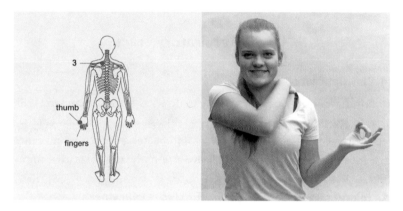

In the case of fever, you can supplement this by also holding the calves—this is what you might call a Jin Shin leg compress.

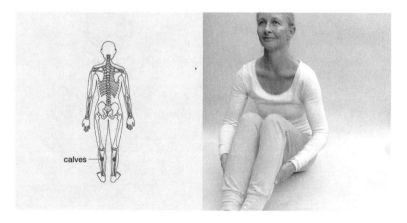

Head Cold

Place one hand on SEL 11 and SEL 3 and the other on SEL 15.

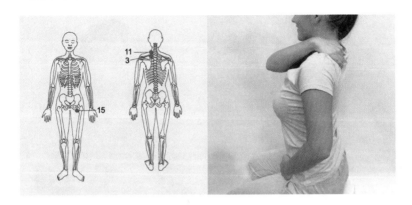

Or hold both SELs 21 by placing your hands under your cheekbones.

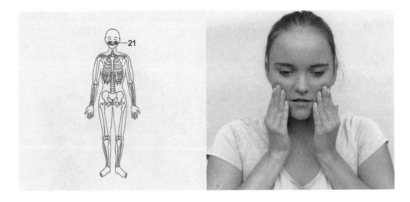

Likewise, SEL 21 held together with SEL 2 frees up the airways.

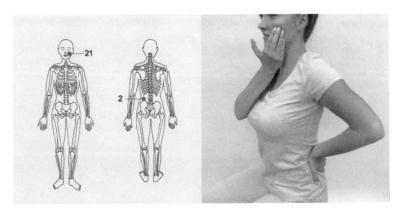

Sinusitis

Hold SEL 21 and SEL 22 on the affected side of the body.

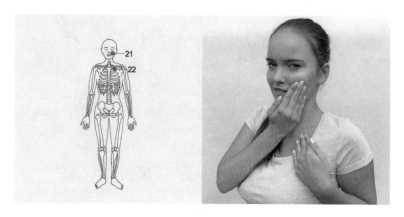

Or place one hand on the forehead on both SELs 20 and the other hand on the back of the neck on both SELs 4.

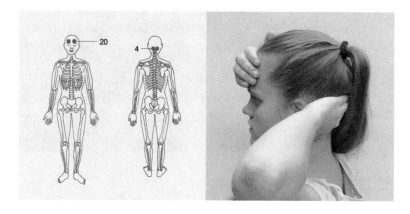

Or use the stomach flow (p. 63).

Throat

Throat Infection and Hoarseness

Place one hand on SEL 11 on the affected side of the body and the other on SEL 13 on the other side of the body.

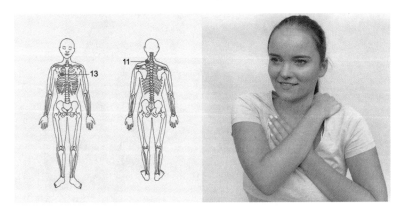

Or place one hand on SEL 11 and SEL 3 on the affected side of the body and form a ring with **thumb and index finger** of the other hand by placing the tip of the thumb on the index-finger nail.

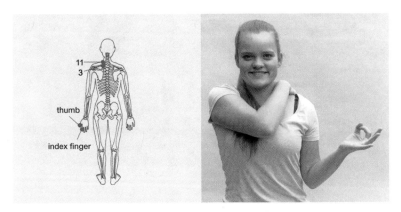

Or use the **stomach flow** (p. 63).

Lower Respiratory Tract

Cough and Bronchitis

Hold the high SEL 19 on the one side of the body and SEL 22 on the other side.

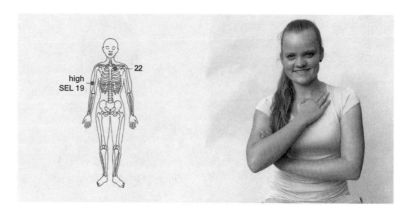

Or hold both SELs 19.

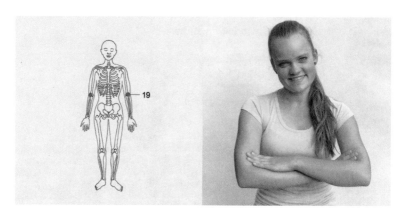

Coughing Fits

You can relieve coughing fits by holding both high SELs 19 (on the backs of the arms).

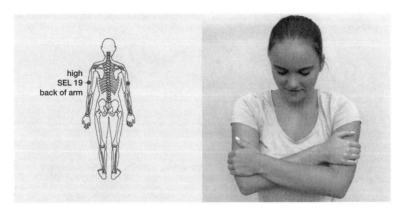

Pneumonia

Pneumonia is not to be trifled with; be sure to get it medically checked.

To strengthen the lungs, you can hold SEL 14 together with SEL 22.

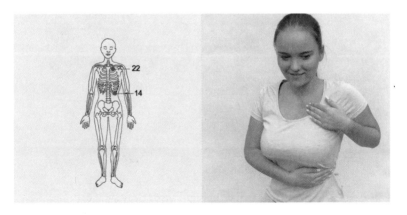

Or hold SEL 3 (the so-called antibiotic hold) together with SEL 15 (p. 78).

Hold the ring finger as often as possible (p. 48).

Respiratory Issues

SEL 1 helps with exhalation and SEL 2 with inhalation. To harmonize breathing, hold SEL 1 together with SEL 2.

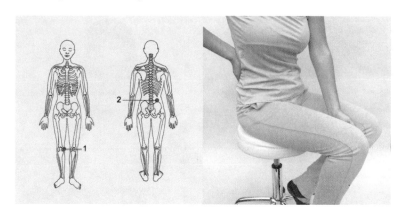

Or hold the high SEL 1 on one side of the body and the high SEL 19 on the other side.

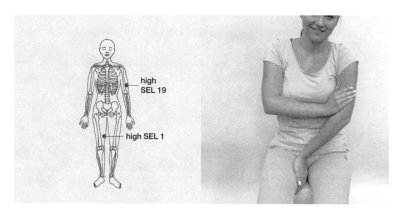

Likewise, the big hug (p. 41) and the supervisor flows (p. 56) bring breathing back into harmony.

Sudden Shortness of Breath

Place one hand on the sternum and the other hand on the top center of the head.

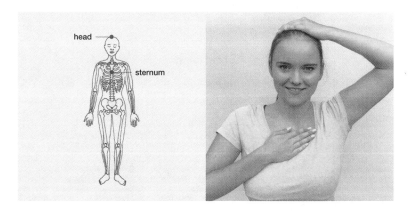

Or place one hand on the upper back of the neck on both SELs 4, and form a ring with thumb and ring finger of the other hand by placing the tip of the thumb on the ring-finger nail.

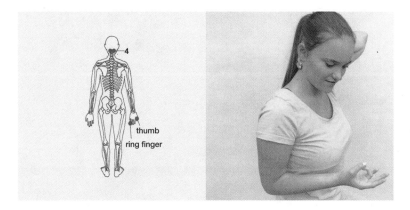

Digestive Organs

Stomach

The stomach flow (p. 63) is suitable for all stomach-related issues.

Stomach Pain

In addition to the stomach flow (p. 63), you can hold both SELs 1.

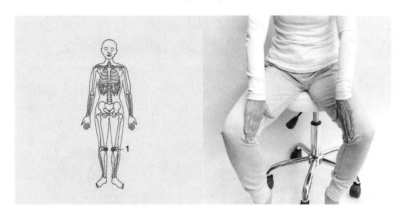

Or hold the high SEL 1 together with the low SEL 8.

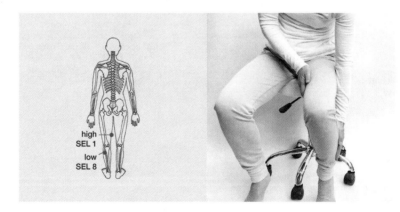

Nausea and Vomiting

Hold both SELs 1 (p. 100). Or place one hand on SEL 1 on one side of the body and the other hand on SEL 14 on the other side.

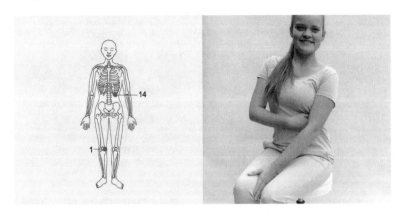

Heartburn

For the left side of the body:

Place your right hand on the left SEL 21 and your left hand on the left SEL 22.

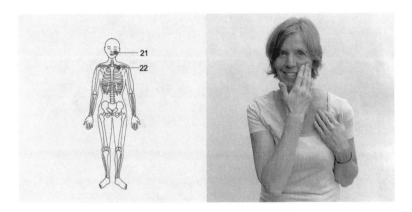

And vice versa for the right side of the body:

Place the left hand on the right SEL 21 and the right hand on the right SEL 22.

You can also hold both SELs 14.

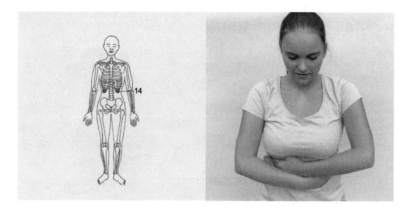

Or place one hand on SEL 14 on one side of the body and the other hand on the high SEL 1 on the other side.

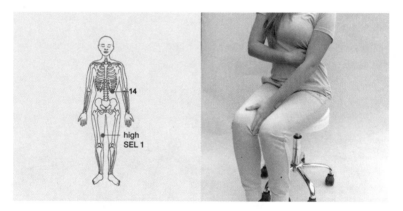

Appetite and Eating Disorders

The spleen flow (p. 59) harmonizes our appetite and eating habits. You can use it for lack of appetite, excessive cravings and eating disorders.

The stomach flow (p. 63) also brings our appetite and weight into balance.

Intestine

Constipation

If constipated, remember to drink enough water and to get enough exercise.

You can also hold SEL 1 (p. 100). Or make a ring with thumb and index finger by placing the tip of the thumb onto the index-finger nail. Place the other hand on SEL 11 (p. 104).

Diarrhea

It is vital to have persistent diarrhea checked by a doctor!

If you have diarrhea, hold both SELs 8.

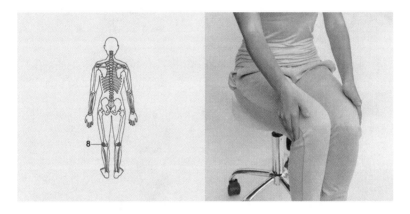

Or place one hand on the right high SEL 1 and the other hand on the right SEL 8.

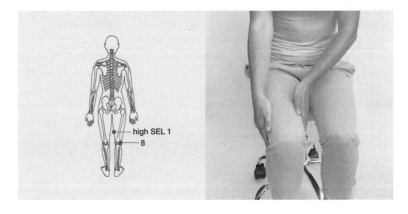

Irritable Bowel

The following is an important hold to soothe intestinal tissue:

Place one hand on the high SEL 1 on one side of the body and the other hand on the high SEL 19 on the other side.

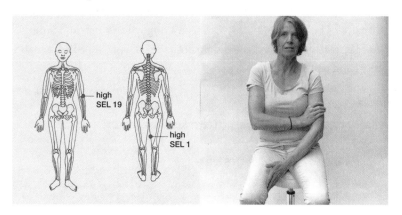

Or make a ring with thumb and index finger of one hand by placing the tip of the thumb on the index-finger nail. Place the other hand on SEL 11.

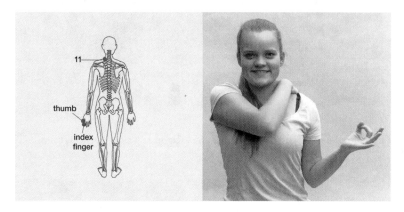

Hemorrhoids

Place one hand on the anal region and the other hand on the SEL 8 on one and then the other side of the body.

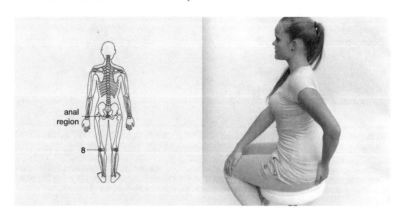

Or hold SEL 14 together with SEL 15.

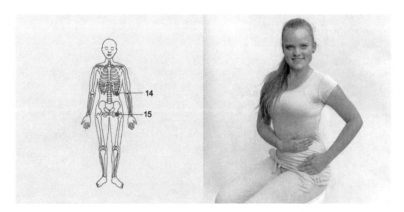

Parasites

For support with treating all types of parasites, hold both SELs 19 (p. 35).

Pancreas

To harmonize the pancreas, hold both SELs 14 (p. 32).

Or place one hand on the left SEL 14 and the other on the left SEL 22.

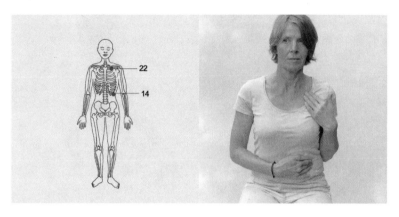

Liver and Gall Bladder

To strengthen the liver, place one hand on the left SEL 4 and the other hand on the right SEL 22.

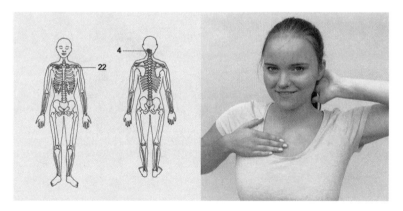

To strengthen the gall bladder, place the right hand on the left SEL 12 and the left hand on the right SEL 20 (see illustrations on next page).

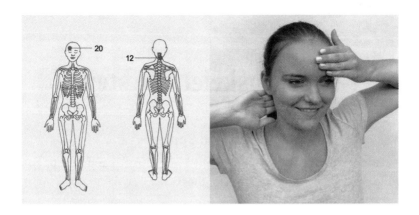

To detox and reduce acidity, place one hand on **SEL 12** and the other hand on **SEL 14**.

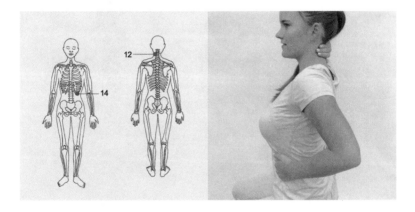

Or hold **SEL 23** together with **SEL 25**.

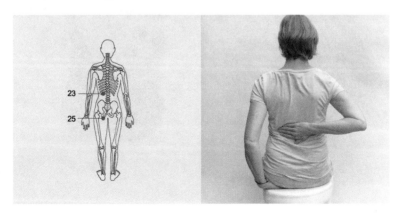

Musculoskeletal System

Back and Spine

The bladder flow (p. 68), the main central flow (p. 52) and the supervisor flows (p. 56) are all important flows for the back.

Your personal Jin Shin chiropractors are SEL 2 and SEL 6.
First hold both SELs 2, then both SELs 6.

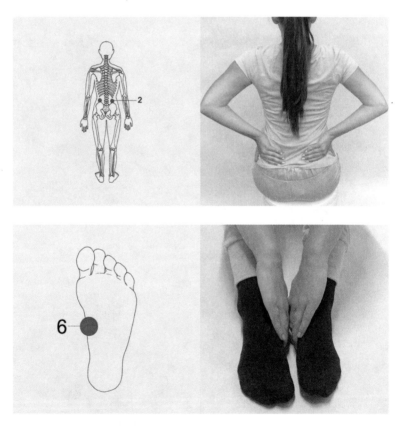

Or hold SEL 2 together with SEL 6.

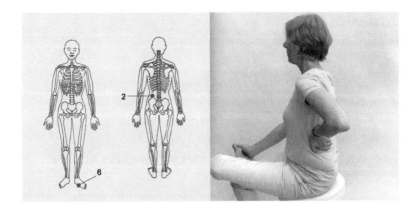

SEL 2 held together with SEL 15 also harmonizes back complaints.

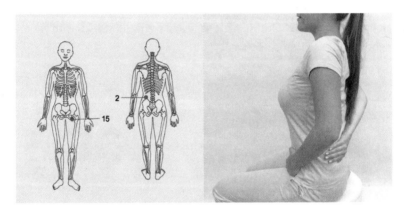

Easiest to perform on yourself is likely the following alternative:
Place your hands in the groin area on **both SELs 15**.

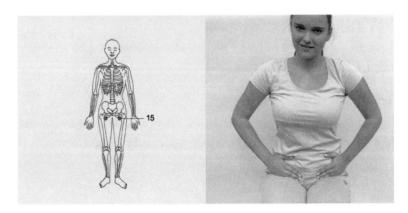

Spinal Disc Issues

An important and very helpful flow for all disc issues is the finger–toe flow (p. 50).

To reduce stress, use the main central flow regularly (p. 52).

Hold your index finger on a regular basis (p. 46) to support the entire back, and the ring finger (p. 48) to support the connective tissue.

Harmonize the supervisor flows (p. 56).

And, if it is comfortable for you, frequently hold both SELs 2 (p. 21).

For spinal disc issues related to the fourth and fifth lumbar vertebrae, do the following:

For the right side of the body:
Hold the left SEL 12 with your left hand and the right SEL 20 with your right hand.

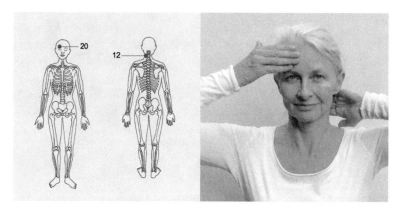

For the left side of the body:
Hold the right SEL 12 with your right hand and the left SEL 20 with your left hand.

Muscles

The following holds support the muscles, balance out muscle tone and help with overexertion, strains, muscle pain, tension and sore muscles:

STEP 1: First place both hands in the hollows of the knees.

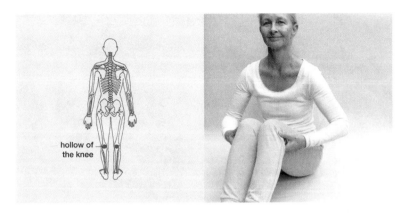

STEP 2: Then place both hands on the upper part of the calves.

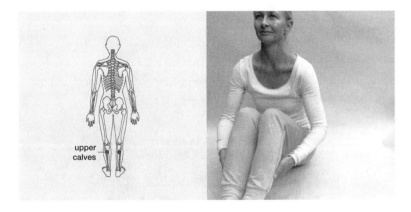

STEP 3: Place both hands on the lower part of the calves.

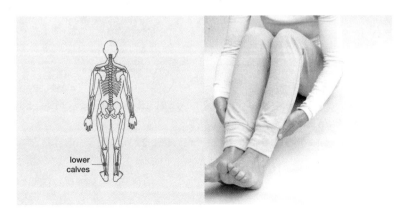

Or hold SEL 5 and SEL 16 with one hand and SEL 8 with the other hand.

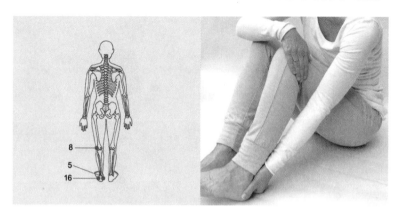

To strengthen weak muscles, hold SEL 12 on one side of the body and SEL 20 on the other side (p. 164).

Ligaments, Tendons, and Joints

For a sprained ankle, simply hold the wrist on the other side of the body. Alternatively, with a sprain place one hand on the affected area and the other hand on the SEL 15 on the same side of the body.

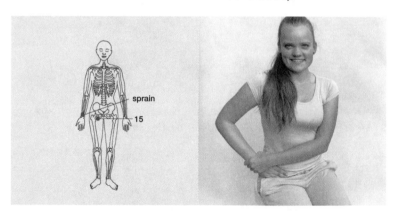

To strengthen ligaments and tendons, hold SEL 12 on one side of the body and SEL 20 on the other side (p. 164).

Or put one hand on SEL 4 and the other on SEL 22 on the same side of the body.

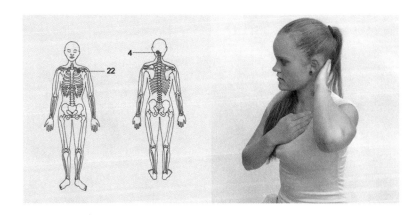

Joint Inflammation (Arthritis)

Regularly use the two detox holds (p. 107).

To relieve pain and heal inflammation, hold SEL 5 and SEL 16 with one hand and place the other hand on SEL 3—it makes no difference whether on the same or opposite side of the body.

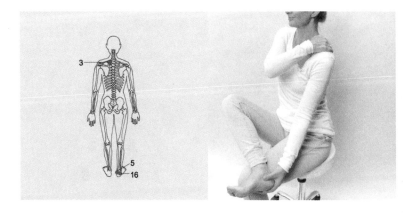

Joint Abrasion (Osteoarthritis)

Hold SEL 13 together with SEL 17.

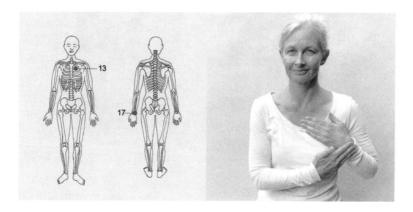

SEL 1 brings movement and agility, so repeatedly hold both SELs 1 (p. 100). Or hold SEL 1 on one side of the body and SEL 19 on the other side.

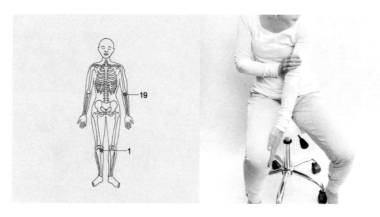

Hip Joint Arthrosis

For the left hip:

Place the left hand on the left SEL 12 and the right hand on the right SEL 20 (p. 107).

And vice versa for the right hip:

Place the right hand on the right SEL 12 and the left hand on the left SEL 20.

Bones

Broken Bones

For healing support with fractures, hold both SELs 15 (p. 32) by placing your hands in the groin area.

Or hold SEL 15 together with SEL 3 on the affected side of the body.

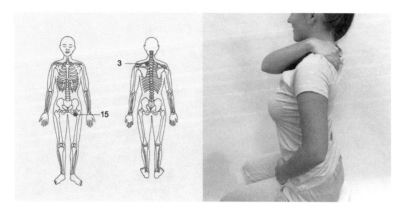

How to Strengthen Your Bones

To fundamentally strengthen the bones, hold SEL 11 on one side of the body and SEL 13 on the other side.

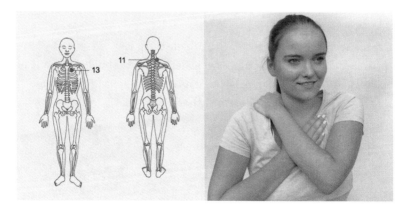

Skin and Hair

The stomach flow (p. 63) is the skin and hair specialist.
The spleen flow (p. 59) also harmonizes the skin.

The calf is also a skin specialist, so hold your calves frequently.

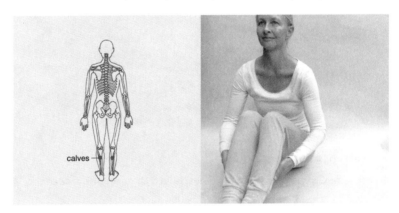

Hair Loss

Use the stomach flow regularly (p. 63) or just step 1.
An over-acidic body often causes hair issues, so use the holds for reducing acidity (p. 107). To harmonize the hormonal system, hold SEL 14 on one side of the body and SEL 22 on the other side.

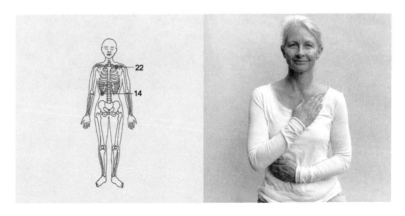

For very thin hair, hair loss or early baldness, place one hand on SEL 11 and hold SEL 17 with the other.

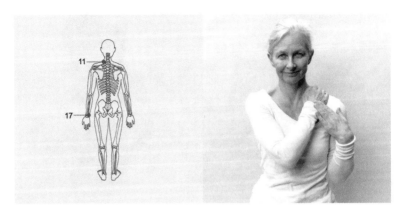

Skin Eczema

Skin issues can have a variety of causes, so always keep an eye on the overall context.

> For general harmonization, regularly use the main central flow (p. 52) and/ or the supervisor flows (p. 56).
> Hold SEL 14 together with SEL 22.

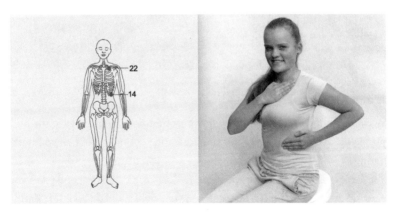

Or hold SEL 3 on one side of the body and SEL 19 on the other side.

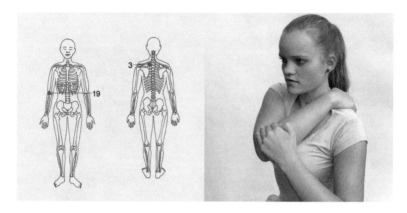

SEL 3 held together with SEL 4 relieves itching.

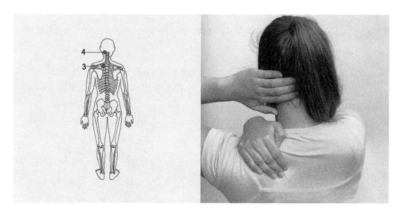

Boils and Abscesses

With boils and abscesses, and whenever something needs to leave the body, place your left hand on the **affected area** and your right hand on your **left hand**.

If there are several people with you, you can also create a "hand pile": you place your left hand on the **abscess** and your right hand on your **left hand**, the next person puts their left hand on your **right hand** and their right hand on their **left hand**, etc. This speeds up the healing process.

Urinary System

Bladder

For all bladder complaints, harmonize the bladder flow (p. 68).

Or hold your index finger (p. 46).
Or hold the backs of your knees.

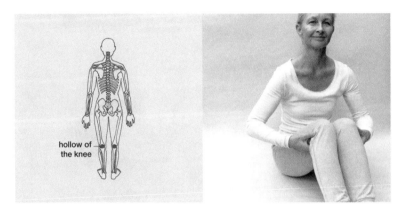

Or hold SEL 23 and SEL 25—either together (as in diagram and photo) or first both SELs 23 and then both SELs 25. If it is easier, you can also hold SEL 23 with the back of the hand.

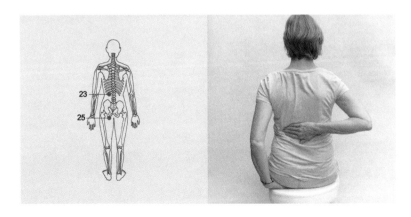

Or place one hand on the **back of the neck** and the other hand on the coccyx.

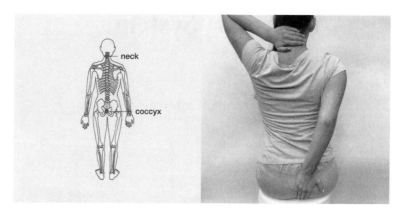

You can also hold SEL 4 together with SEL 13.

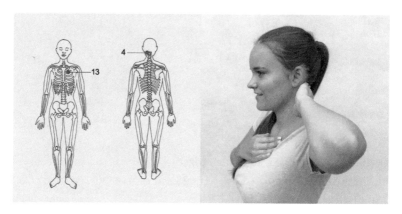

Kidneys

Kidney inflammation can be treated as follows:

For the right side of the body:

STEP 1: First hold the right SEL 3 together with the right SEL 15.

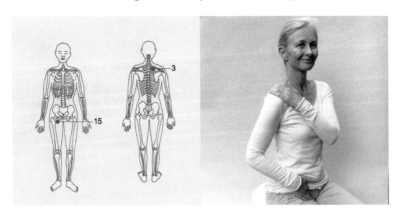

STEP 2: Then place one hand on the pubic bone and hold the right little toe with the other hand.

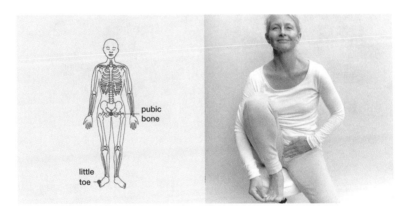

And vice versa for the left side of the body:

STEP 1: Hold the left SEL 3 and the left SEL 15.

STEP2: Then place one hand on the pubic bone and hold the left little toe with the other hand.

Kidney and Bladder Stones

Hold SEL 5 and SEL 16 with one hand and place the other hand on SEL 23.

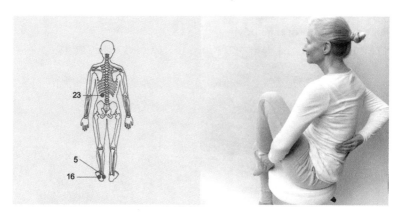

Or hold SEL 23 and SEL 14.

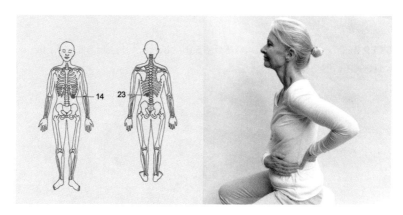

Genital Organs

Male Genital Organs

Testicular Inflammation

Hold SEL 3 with one hand and SEL 15 on the affected side of the body with the other hand.

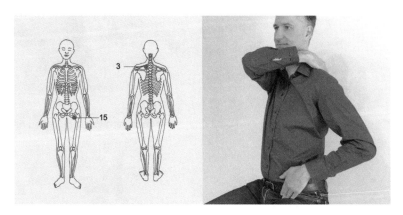

Prostate

To strengthen the prostate, use the spleen flow (p. 59).
Or place one hand on the sternum and the other on the coccyx.

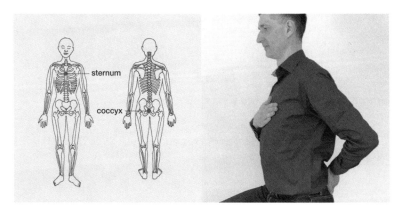

Female Genital Organs

Menstrual Cramps

Place one hand on SEL 4 on one side of the body and the other hand on SEL 13 on the other side.

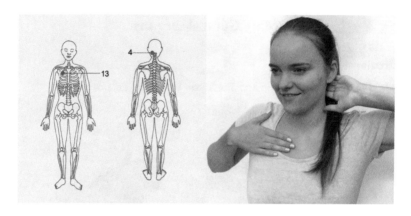

Or put one hand on SEL 13 on one side of the body and the other hand on SEL 15 on the other side.

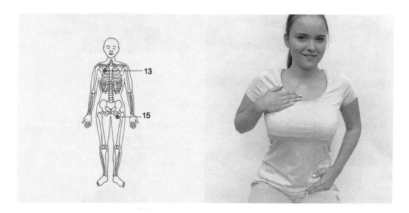

Inflammation of Ovaries and Cysts

Use the spleen flow (p. 59).

Or place your hands, with your arms crossed, on both SELs 13 (p. 31).

Pregnancy and Birth

Pregnancy

Holding both SELs 22 (p. 37) together will help you adapt to this new situation. It also helps the unborn baby to develop in the best possible way.

The main central flow (p. 52) is also a great flow for mother and child. As it connects mind and matter, it supports the child's mental, psychological and physical development and also gives the mother confidence and energy.

Morning Sickness

Hold both SELs 1 with arms crossed (p. 20).
Or hold your wrist with one hand and form a ring with thumb and middle finger with the other hand by placing the tip of your thumb on the middle-finger nail.

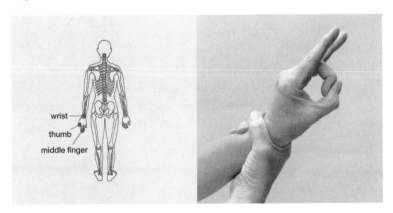

Fatigue and Exhaustion

SEL 25 is located at the lower end of the sitting bone (p. 40).
Sitting on your hands helps to recharge depleted energy batteries and regain vitality and life force.
Holding the high SEL 1 on one side of the body and the high SEL 19 on the other side helps in regaining momentum.

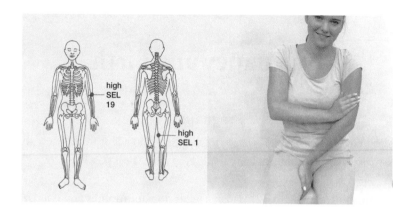

Or place one hand on the back of the neck and the other hand on the coccyx (p. 120).

Preparation for Birth

If the baby does not want to turn into the birth position, you can support it by using the bladder flow (p. 68).

SEL 8 (p. 27) softens the pelvis and opens it for birth.

SEL 22 relaxes and helps mother and baby to prepare for birth. Hold both SELs 22 (p. 37) with arms crossed.

Birth Support

Also during birth, it can be great to treat yourself—or better yet, to receive a treatment. SEL 4 together with SEL 13 relaxes, brings about confidence and calm and promotes a swift birth.

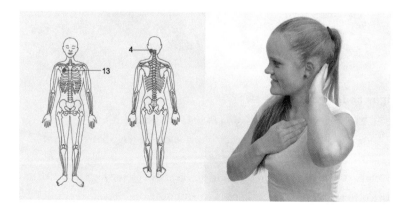

Both SELs 11 help to release tensions and stress.

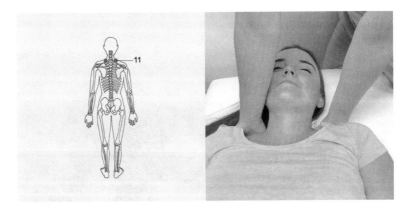

If you are treating yourself, hold SEL 11 together with SEL 15 (p. 30). It is also very comforting and supportive to hold the sacrum together with SEL 8.

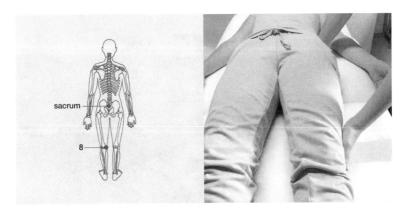

If the contractions are severe and the pain overwhelming, let someone hold both SELs 5 together with both SELs 16 for you (p. 157).
For fear and panic hold your index finger (p. 46).

The Newborn

SEL 4 supports breathing, so place one hand on both SELs 4 and the other hand on the coccyx.

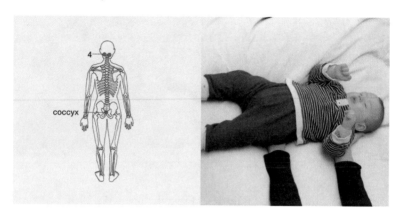

If your baby is born with an illness, disability or weakness, hold both SELs 1 daily for one year. This will help the child develop in the best possible way.

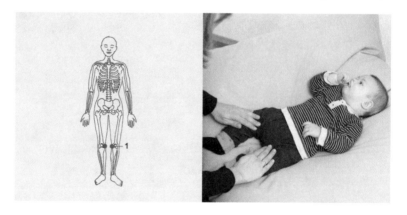

The following hold strengthens the baby all over and allows for the best start to a healthy and strong life:

Place one hand on the shoulder blades in the area of SEL 9 and SEL 26 and the other hand on the lower back in the area of SEL 2.

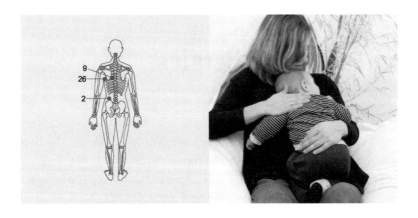

If your baby vomits often or is prone to stomach ache, hold both SELs 1 (p. 100). You can also place a hand on one SEL 1 while breastfeeding.

Breast Infection

The spleen flow (p. 59) is an important flow for the days following delivery and for the duration of breastfeeding. It helps regulate the production of milk and aids with breast infection.

Also hold both SELs 13.

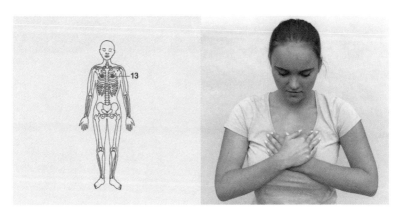

Allergies

Allergies are a widespread issue and can have a variety of causes. The harmonization and stabilization of the immune system (p. 136) is important and of course the psycho-emotional background as to why the body reacts defensively to certain stimuli that it should simply accept.

An important energy lock for intolerances of all kinds is SEL 22.

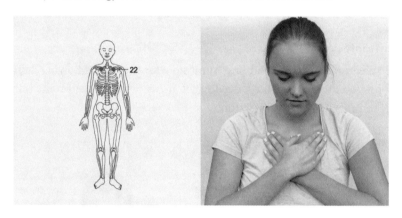

Also, high SEL 19, located about a hand's breadth above SEL 19, is an important point for all allergies. With arms crossed, hold the insides of your upper arms, moving your fingertips a little towards the backs of the arms, where a point that is sensitive to pain can often be felt.

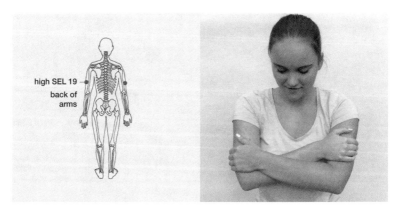

If the airways are affected, place one hand on SEL 22 and the other hand on SEL 14, first on one side of the body and then on the other side.

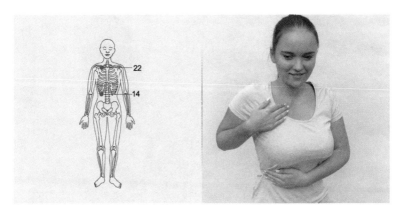

Or hold **both SELs 1** with arms crossed (p. 20).

Or place one hand on the **high SEL 1 on one side** of the body and the other hand on **SEL 19 on the other side.**

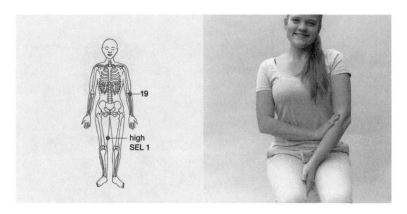

In cases of **food allergies**, use the **stomach flow** (p. 63).

Or hold **SEL 11** with one hand on one side of the body and **SEL 13** with the other hand on the other side.

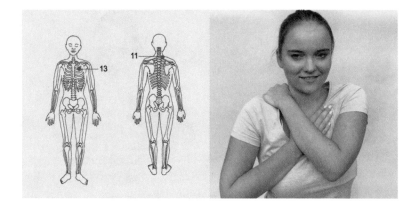

If the **skin** is affected, the **stomach flow** (p. 63) and the **spleen flow** (p. 59) work well.

The **main central flow** (p. 52) and the **mediator flows** (p. 58) also provide support in this instance.

Nervous System

Neuralgia

For neuralgia in the head region, use the stomach flow (p. 63).

For pain relief, hold SEL 5 together with SEL 16 (p. 24).
Or hold SEL 17 (p. 34).

Muscle Twitching

Muscle twitching can accompany various neurological conditions. These include disorders in the nervous system as well as in the nerve cells of the muscular system. Be sure to have this condition checked by a doctor. Muscle twitching is not always based on an illness and is often harmless. Sometimes a temporary nerve irritation may also cause this symptom.

Hold SEL 8 together with SEL 17.

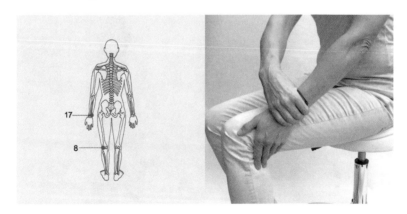

Paralysis

In cases of paralysis of any kind, use the following holds in turn:

For the right side of the body:

STEP 1: Place the right hand on the right SEL 4 and the left hand on the right SEL 13.

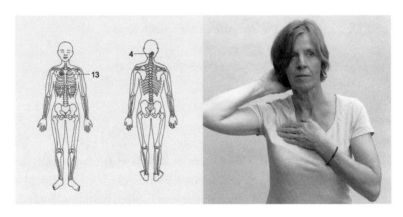

STEP 2: Then place the right hand on the right SEL 15 and the left hand on the right SEL 16.

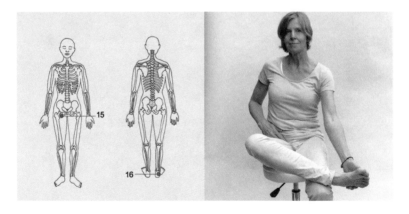

And vice versa for the left side of the body:

STEP 1: Place the left hand on the left SEL 4 and the right hand on the left SEL 13.

STEP 2: Then place the left hand on the left SEL 15 and the right hand on the left SEL 16.

Epilepsy

SEL 7 is an important energy lock for epilepsy. You can also hold it together with SEL 24, since the two energy locks support each other well.

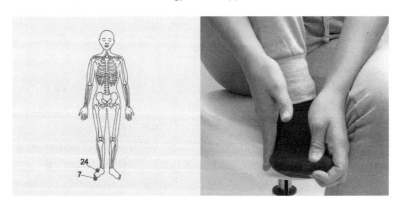

Hold the back of the neck and forehead frequently.

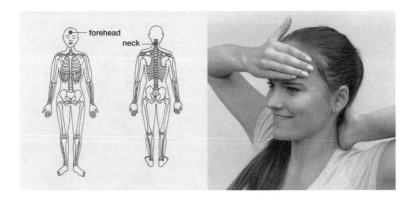

Hold SEL 12 with SEL 14 repeatedly.

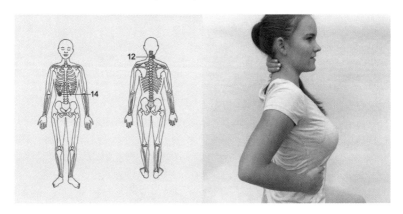

Immune System

An intact immune system is a prerequisite for health and vitality. As soon as you start treating yourself, your immune system will be automatically strengthened and self-healing processes set in motion.

Of course, there are also special flows or holds to activate the immune system. The most important energy lock for a well-functioning immune system is SEL 3. It is, so to speak, the door through which viruses and bacteria can leave the body. When this door swings open, old, used-up energy can be discharged and new, purified energy can be let in.

SEL 15 supports SEL 3, so it is best to hold these two energy locks together.

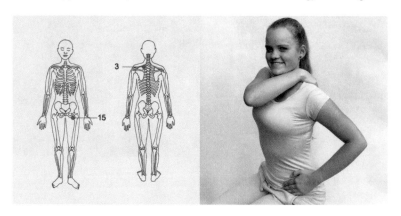

Other important flows for harmonizing the immune system are:

- the main central flow (p. 52),
- the supervisor flows (p. 56),
- and the spleen flow (p. 59).

You can also hold both SELs 19 together with both high SELs 19.

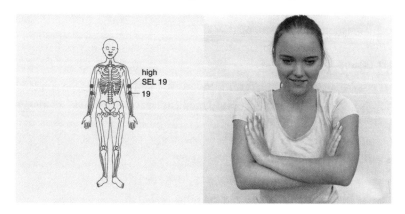

Cardiovascular System

To strengthen the cardiovascular system, hold all fingers (p. 44) one at a time. Also use the big hug (p. 41).

Heart Issues

Heart issues can be life-threatening and must, in all instances, be treated by a doctor. Needless to say, in addition to medical treatment, flows can always be supportive. Hold your little finger repeatedly (p. 49).

Pressure in the Heart Area and Anxiety

Place your hands on the groin area on both SELs 15 (p. 32).
Or place one hand on SEL 15 and the other on SEL 6.

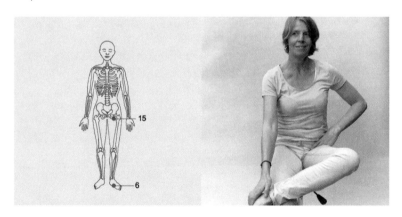

Rapid Heartbeat

Hold SEL 14 on one side of the body together with the high SEL 19 on the other side.

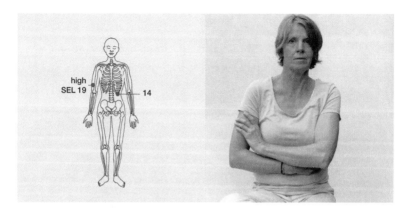

Irregular Heartbeat

Hold SEL 17 (p. 34).

Or hold SEL 17 on one side of the body and SEL 11 on the other side.

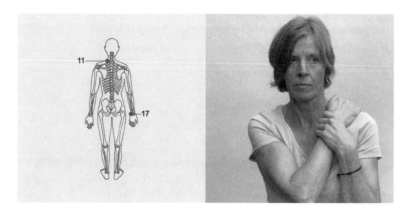

Blood Pressure

To harmonize low or high blood pressure, hold both high SELs 19 (p. 35). Or hold both SELs 2 (p. 21).

Or place one hand on the back of the neck and the other hand on the coccyx (p. 120).

SEL 23 held together with SEL 25 also regulates blood pressure. If it is easier, you can also hold SEL 23 with the back of the hand.

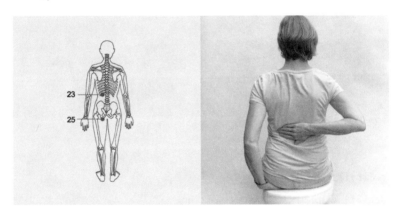

Circulatory Issues

For circulatory issues, hold both high SELs 19 (p. 35).

Or hold SEL 17 (p. 34). SEL 17 is also an important energy lock if you faint easily or in cases of circulatory collapse.

To stabilize circulation, also hold SEL 22 together with SEL 23.

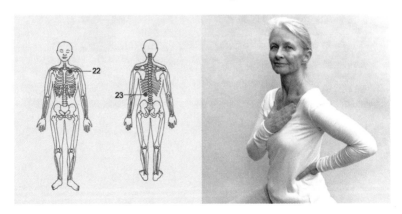

Place one hand on the back of the neck on both SELs 4 and the other on the forehead on both SELs 20.

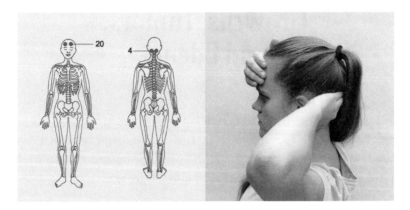

You can also stabilize circulation by placing one hand on the sternum and the other on the coccyx.

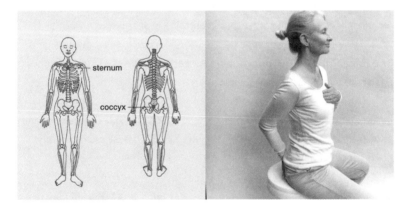

Growths, Tumors, and Edema

Where there is movement, accumulation cannot set in. Treatments bring energy flows back into motion, so that what is old and hardened can be released. Jin Shin Jyutsu harmonizes the whole being and gradually brings everything back into balance —including also cell growth.

SEL 1 (p. 100), the primary mover, sets everything in motion and dissolves congestion and accumulation.

Regularly use the main central flow (p. 52) and the big hug (p. 41) to fully reconnect to source and trust that everything is possible.

The spleen flow (p. 59) brings light into each cell and can dissolve tumors and accumulations.

In turn, hold the left SEL 20 together with the right SEL 19 (diagram and photo) and the right SEL 20 with the left SEL 19. These are important holds for cell renewal!

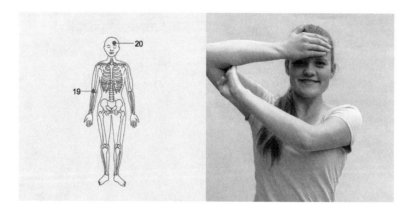

Regularly use the supervisor flows (p. 56).

To detox and reduce acidity in the body hold SEL 23 and SEL 25 (p. 107). Or hold SEL 11 and with the other hand form a ring with thumb and index finger by placing the tip of the thumb on the index-finger nail.

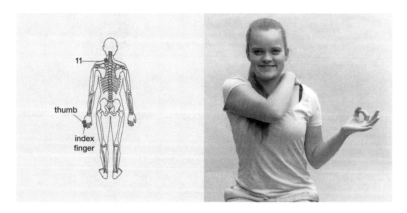

An important hold for malignant tumors is as follows:

Put one hand on SEL 24 (harmonizes chaos) and the other hand on SEL 26.

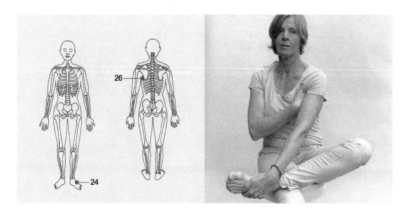

For lumps and cysts in the chest, place one hand under the armpit of the affected side of the body, with the thumb pointing up (as in the big hug, p. 41) and the other hand on the high SEL 1 on the other side of the body.

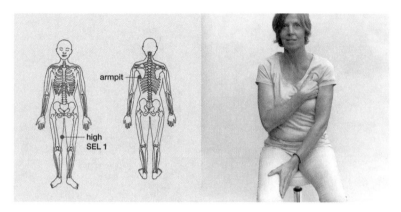

If the hand is uncomfortable under the armpit, place it on the outside of the upper arm near the armpit instead.

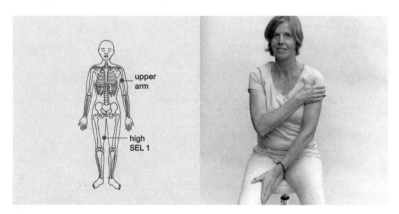

The bladder flow (p. 68) harmonizes the balance of fluids and can dissolve edema.

Injuries and Emergencies

Wounds

For bleeding wounds, place your right hand on or over the wound or wound dressing and the left hand on the right hand.

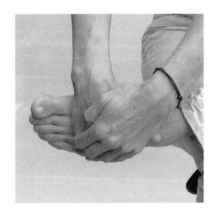

For festering wounds, place the left hand on or over the wound or wound dressing and the right hand on the left hand.

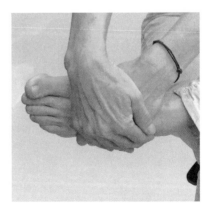

If you want to treat yourself but the wound is in a location that you cannot reach with both hands, e.g., a hand, simply place one hand on or over the affected area.

Hematoma

Cross your hands so that your little fingers touch. In this position, place them on the affected area.

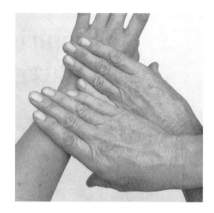

If you want to treat yourself, but the hematoma is in a location that you cannot reach with both hands, e.g., a hand, simply place one hand on the affected area.

Stings, Splinters, and Thorns

Place the left hand on or over the affected area and the right hand on the left hand (p. 145).

If you want to treat yourself, but the sting, splinter or thorn is in a location that you cannot reach with both hands, e.g., a hand, simply place one hand on the affected area.

Burns

Place both hands next to each other onto or over the affected area.

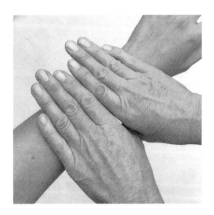

If you want to treat yourself, but the burn is in a location that you cannot reach with both hands, eg. a hand, simply place one hand on or over the affected area. Or hold both calves.

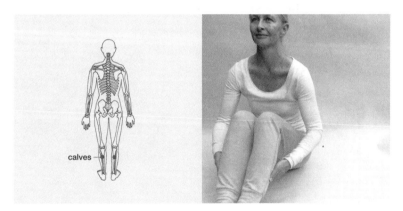

calves

Concussion and Head Injuries

First hold both SELs 4 and then both SELs 7.

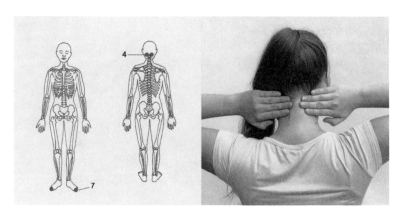

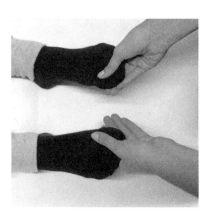

If you have trouble holding both SELs 7, let someone else treat you.

Bone Fractures

For healing support with fractures, hold both SELs 15 by placing your hands in the groin area.

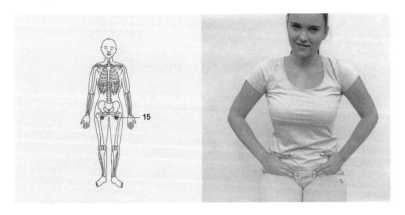

Or hold SEL 15 together with SEL 3 on the affected side of the body.

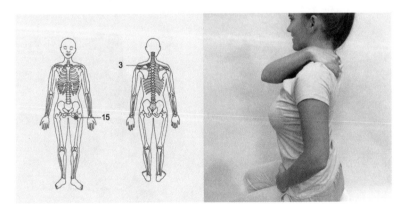

Bruises

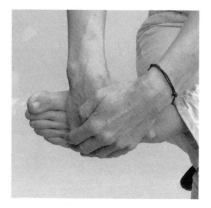

Place the right hand on the affected area and the left hand on the right hand. Or place one hand on the affected area.

Sprains

For a sprained ankle, hold the wrist on the other side of the body. Alternatively, for a sprain place one hand on the affected area and the other hand on SEL 15 on the same side of the body.

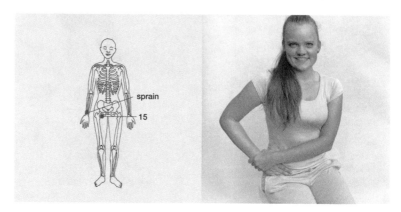

Shock

Shock is a life-threatening condition of the circulatory system and always needs to be checked by a doctor. It can have various causes, e.g., heatstroke, injury, severe blood loss, allergic reaction, poisoning, illness, bacterial infection, etc.

Frightening situations can also cause shock. Signs of shock include: pale and cold skin, rapid and shallow breathing, accelerated heartbeat, cold sweats, feeling cold, shaking, restlessness, anxiety or confusion.

Call an ambulance and treat both SELs 1 until they arrive.

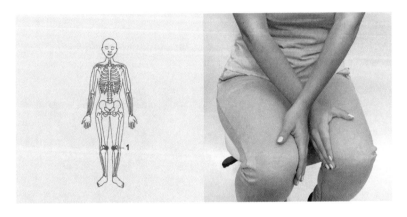

SEL 4 and SEL 7 are emergency points. Hold both SELs 4 on the back of the neck (see below) and both SELs 7 on the undersides of the big toes (see next page).

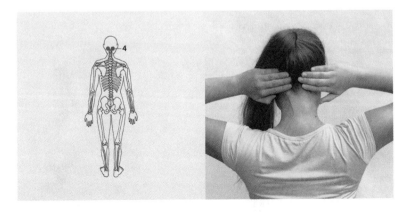

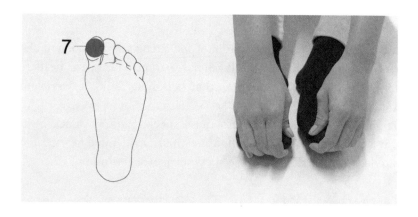

Poisoning

In cases of poisoning a doctor must also be consulted immediately. As a first aid help hold both SELs 1.

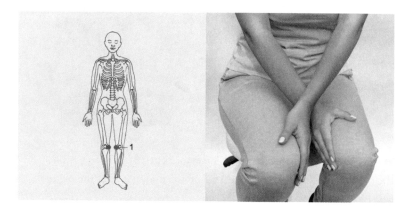

In addition, hold SEL 21 and SEL 23.

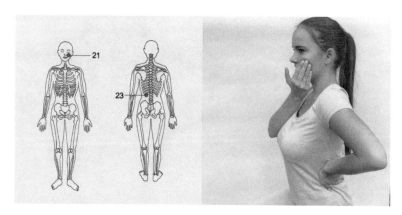

Heatstroke and Sunstroke

The first aid holds for excessive sun or heat are:

Hold both SELs 4.

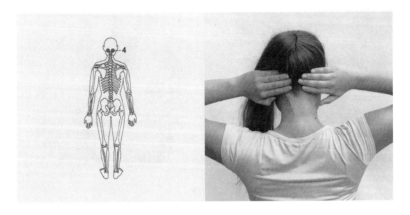

Hold both SELs 7.

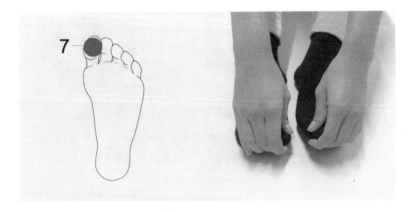

Choking and Shortness of Breath

Hold both SELs 1.

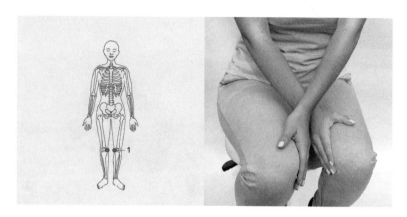

Or hold SEL 1 together with SEL 2.

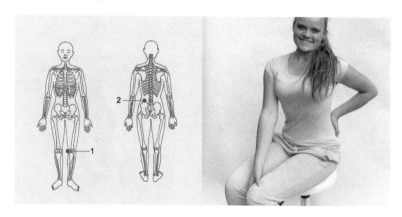

Surgery

Hold both SELs 15 before and after surgeries.

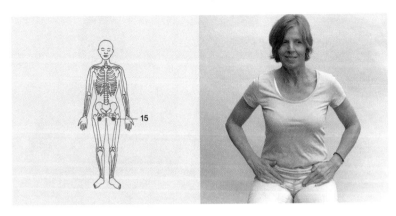

Or hold SEL 15 together with SEL 11.

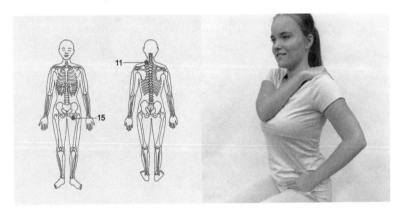

Travel Sickness

Hold both SELs 14.

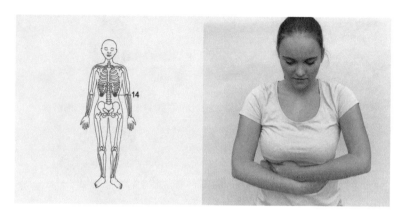

Or hold SEL 14 together with SEL 1.

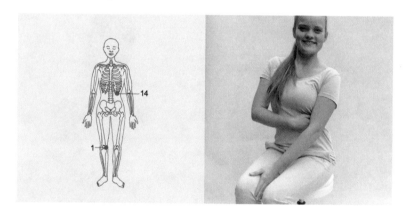

Pain

All kinds of pain can be alleviated by holding SEL 5 together with
SEL 16 (p. 24), first on one side of the body and then on the other side.
If another person treats you, both SELs 5 and both SELs 16 can be held
simultaneously, as shown in the photo.

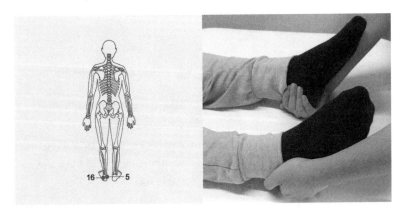

Overexertion

Hold SEL 15 together with SEL 24.

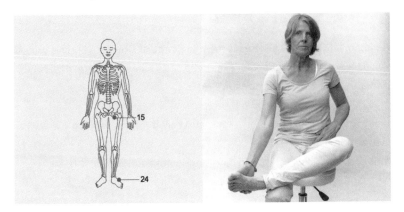

Mental Stress

Fear and Panic

The following is the emergency hold for any anxiety and panic:

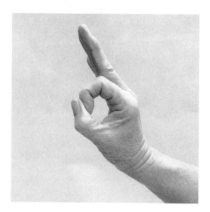

Hold the index finger (p. 46).
Or form a ring with thumb
and index finger by placing the
tip of the thumb on the index-
finger nail.

An important flow for all fears is the main central flow (p. 52). This brings
you back to your center and evokes deep trust. The big hug (p. 41) also
calms you down and helps dissolve fears.

Hold SEL 4 (p. 23). This energy lock, also called "the window to the sky",
evokes primal trust.
SEL 12 (p. 31) helps you feel in harmony—with your origins, with source,
with God—and releases fear and panic.

Important energy locks for the subject of fear are SEL 21, SEL 22 and SEL 23. You can combine these energy locks as follows:

For the left side of the body:

STEP 1: Place your right hand on the left SEL 21 and your left hand on the left SEL 23.

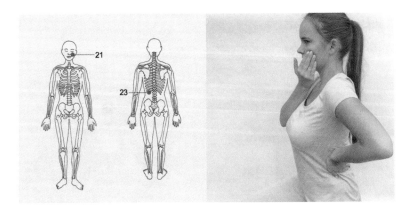

STEP 2: Then leave your left hand on the left SEL 23 and place your right hand on the left SEL 22.

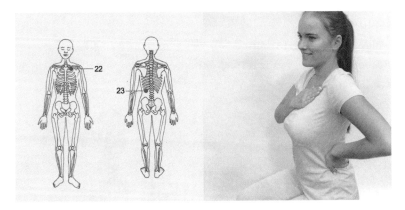

For the right side of the body, reverse the sequence:

STEP 1: First place your left hand on the right SEL 21 and your right hand on the right SEL 23.

STEP 2: The right hand stays on the right SEL 23 and the left hand moves to the right SEL 22.

The bladder flow (p. 68) gives you a sense of inner safety and deep serenity. It helps with panic attacks, fears and phobias. Or place one hand on the sternum and the other hand on the coccyx.

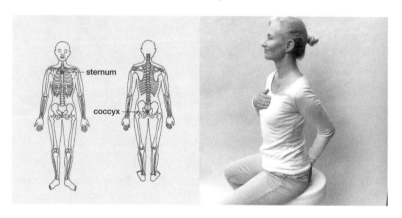

Insecurities

Hold SEL 17 or SEL 18 (both p. 34).

Reinforce your inner strength and authority by holding both SELs 19 in the crook of the arm.

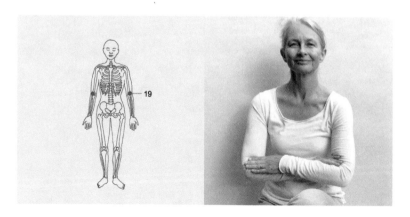

Nervousness and Jumpiness

In this instance, too, the main central flow (p. 52) is a great support. Hold SEL 17 repeatedly during the day.

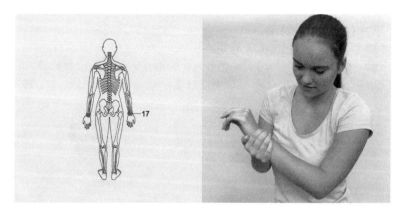

Or hold SEL 21 and SEL 22.

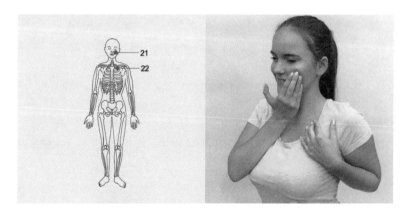

Stress and Tension

Repeatedly use the big hug (p. 41): "Give yourself a big hug. Be the dropping of your shoulders and exhale all dust, dirt and greasy grime." (*M. Burmeister*)

The supervisor flows (p. 56) help release stress and tension. Or hold both SELs 15 (p. 30) or both SELs 25 (p. 40). SEL 2 also releases tension and stress and relaxes the back of the neck, shoulders and back. Hold both SELs 2 (p. 21). Or place one hand on SEL 2 and the other hand on SEL 15.

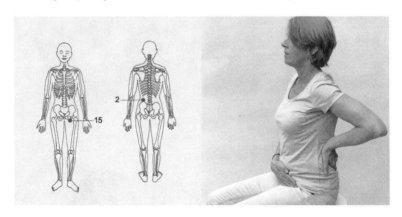

SEL 17 (p. 34) relaxes the mind and nerves.

Homesickness

To relieve homesickness, hold both SELs 19 (p. 35). In addition, you can also hold SEL 11 together with SEL 12.

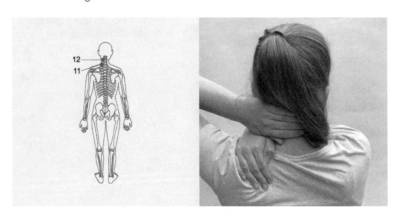

SEL 22 (p. 37) helps you adapt to new situations.

Jealousy

A helpful flow for jealousy is the stomach flow (p. 63).

Or hold SEL 14 together with SEL 24. SEL 24 harmonizes chaos—also on the inner level.

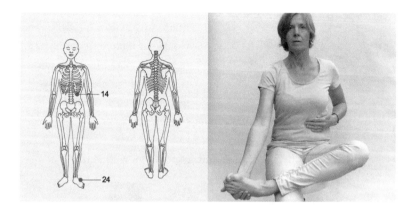

You can also hold SEL 14 together with SEL 22 (p. 97). Or hold SEL 14 on one side of the body with the high SEL 19 on the other side.

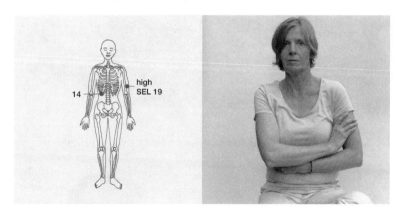

Rage, Anger, and Aggression

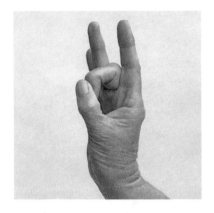

If you have a fundamental issue with managing rage and aggression, ensure good basic harmonization by using the main central flow (p. 52). Hold your middle finger (p. 47) repeatedly. Or form a ring with thumb and middle finger by placing the tip of the thumb on the middle-finger nail.

Hold both SELs 24 (p. 39). Or hold SEL 24 together with SEL 26.

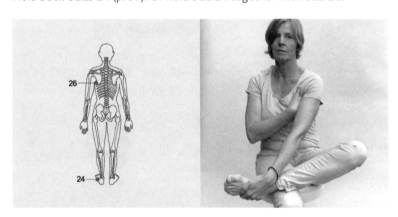

Hold SEL 12 on one side of the body and SEL 20 on the other side.

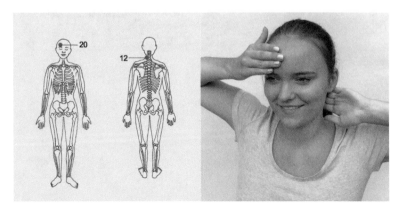

Depletion and Fatigue

Hold both SELs 25 (p. 40) by sitting on your hands. Body, mind and emotions come to rest while you are replenished with new energy.

The following finger position removes tiredness from the body and helps you to relax and refuel:

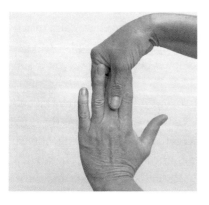

Place your right thumb on the back of the left middle finger and the other right fingers on the front of this finger. Practise the big hug (p. 41).

Insomnia

While trying to fall asleep hold SEL 18 (p. 35). It relaxes you and stops the thoughts from going round in circles. Hold your thumb (p. 45) to help you switch off, fall asleep and deal with nightmares.

The following finger position also harmonizes sleep:

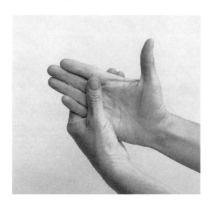

For the left side of the body: Place your right thumb on the front of the left little finger and the ring finger and the other right fingers on the backs of these fingers.

And vice versa for the right side of the body:
Place the left thumb on the front of the right little finger and the ring finger and the other left fingers on the backs of these fingers.

Epilogue

J in Shin Jyutsu is a wonderful way to harmonize life energy and to activate self-healing powers. It can be used anytime, anywhere, and also in parallel to drug treatments or other forms of therapy. As such, it allows you to support yourself and your family in all aspects of life.

Jin Shin Jyutsu is a very gentle method and sometimes it may take a little while to make a noticeable difference. Stay tuned and try out the different flow sequences. Also hold your fingers regularly, one at a time. You can do this, for example, if you have to wait at a traffic light or at the checkout. Make it a habit. In this way, you will gradually strengthen yourself from the inside out. You will see how your immune system, as well as your emotional state, becomes more stable, how you feel stronger, more vital and fulfilled.

With all of my heart I wish you much joy in discovering and experiencing the power and magic of Jin Shin healing touch!

Sincerely,
Tina Stümpfig

Acknowledgements

I thank Jiro Murai for the rediscovery of Jin Shin Jyutsu and for bringing this wonderful healing art back to the world. I thank Mary Burmeister for dedicating her life to this art and for bringing it to the West.

Thank you to all Jin Shin Jyutsu teachers who are spreading this knowledge to make it accessible to ever more people.

I thank my daughter Mira Stümpfig for the illustrations and the models Samaya and Lucia Stümpfig, Bettina von Nottbeck, Miriam Burtscher, Torsten Steppe, Johannes and Ulrike Dehner and Paula and Andrea Haag.

Further Information

Information about the author's courses and seminars can be found at:

www.harmonie-der-mitte.de

For more information about Jin Shin Jyutsu, as well as practitioners and seminars in your area, visit the Jin Shin Jyutsu Europe office:

www.jinshinjyutsu.de

Jin Shin Jyutsu® Physio philosophy is copyrighted in the United States and the proper name of Jin Shin Jyutsu Inc., Scottsdale, Arizona.

Recommended Reading

Burmeister, Alice. *The Touch of Healing*. New York: Bantam Books, 1997.

Burmeister, Mary. *Introducing Jin Shin Jyutsu Is, Books 1–3*. Scottsdale, AZ: Jin Shin Jyutsu, Inc., 1980.

Burmeister, Mary. *What Mary Says: The Wisdom of Mary Burmeister*. Audio edition. Scottsdale, AZ: Jin Shin Jyutsu, Inc., 1997.

Fahrnow, Ilse-Maria. *Mehr Energie mit Jin Shin Jyutsu*. Munich, Germany: Südwest Verlag, 2012.

Riegger-Krause, Waltraud. *Health Is in Your Hands: Jin Shin Jyutsu – Practicing the Art of Self-Healing*. New York: Upper West Side Philosophers, Inc., 2014.

———. *Jin Shin Jyutsu – Einfache Anwendung zur Selbsthilfe*. Munich, Germany: Südwest Verlag, 2005.

Stümpfig-Rüdisser, Tina. *Meine Hände helfen und heilen*. Petersberg, Germany: Verlag Via Nova, 2008.

———. *Jin Shin Jyutsu – Die Heilkraft liegt in Dir*. Petersberg, Germany: Verlag Via Nova, 2009.

———. *Lebensquell Jin Shin Jyutsu*. Petersberg, Germany: Verlag Via Nova, 2010.

———. *Jin Shin Jyutsu – Das Powerprogramm für Kinder und Jugendliche*. Petersberg, Germany: Verlag Via Nova, 2011.

———. *Jin Shin Jyutsu – Die Kunst des Heilströmens erlernen*. Petersberg, Germany: Verlag Via Nova, 2013.

———. *Jin Shin Jyutsu in der Schwangerschaft*. Petersberg, Germany: Verlag Via Nova, 2014.

Index

About the Author

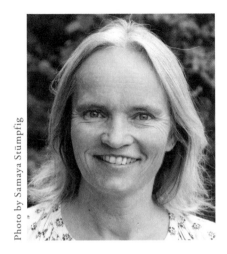

Photo by Samaya Stümpfig

TINA STÜMPFIG, psychologist and special education specialist, has been working as a Jin Shin Jyutsu practitioner with humans and animals for many years. In individual treatments as well as in group seminars, she shows that everything we need to be happy and healthy lies within ourselves. She has already written several textbooks on the subject of Jin Shin Jyutsu.

For more information visit: **www.harmonie-der-mitte.de**

FINDHORN PRESS

Life-Changing Books

Learn more about us and our books at
www.findhornpress.com

For information on the Findhorn Foundation:
www.findhorn.org